CW00494161

Children of the Cure

Missing Data, Lost Lives and Antidepressants

David Healy

Joanna Le Noury

Julie Wood

Samizdat Health

Samizdat Health Writer's Co-operative Inc.

Cover Design/Illustration: Billiam James, image adapted from *Adam and Eve* by Lucas Cranach the Elder

First Printing, 2020

Title: Children of the Cure: Missing Data, Lost Lives and Antidepressants

ISBN: 978-1-7770565-6-8

Publisher: Samizdat Health Writer's Co-operative Inc.

www.samizdathealth.org
www.study329.org
www.davidhealy.org

Dedication

There are some people closely linked to the authors to whom Children of the Cure is dedicated including John David Wood, Shane Clancy, Sarah Carlin, Stephen O'Neill, Jake McGill Lynch, Woody Witzcak, Natalie Gehrki, Candace Downing, Brennan McCartney.

Others who became the victims of violence caused by SSRIs like the 12 people who died at a Batman movie in Aurora Colorado, and Rita Schell and Deborah and Alyssa Tobin who died in Gillette Wyoming. This is a growing list.

There are many others whose lives were badly disrupted by SSRIs but who in some cases have turned the harms into public health advances like Anne Marie Kelly, Annie Bevan, Katinka Newman, Bob Fiddaman, Leonie Fennel, and Colleen Bell.

Lyam Kilker and all the children who miscarried, died because of birth defects, or live with birth defects—another growing list.

Young people who have taken their own lives or sought assisted dying because of enduring withdrawal syndromes or Post-SSRI Sexual Dysfunction (PSSD), of whom David Stofkooper is the best known but there are others.

People who have died by suicide, homicide, or suffered other serious injuries following over 200 different non-psychotropic drugs such as doxycycline, isotretinoin, finasteride, and the fluoroquinolone antibiotics.

The children who participated in Study 329 who have never been told the truth about what happened to them – and the tens of thousands of others, children, elderly, and disadvantaged in one way or the other who are fed through trials and injured without any acknowledgment.

The book is also dedicated to Mickey Nardo.

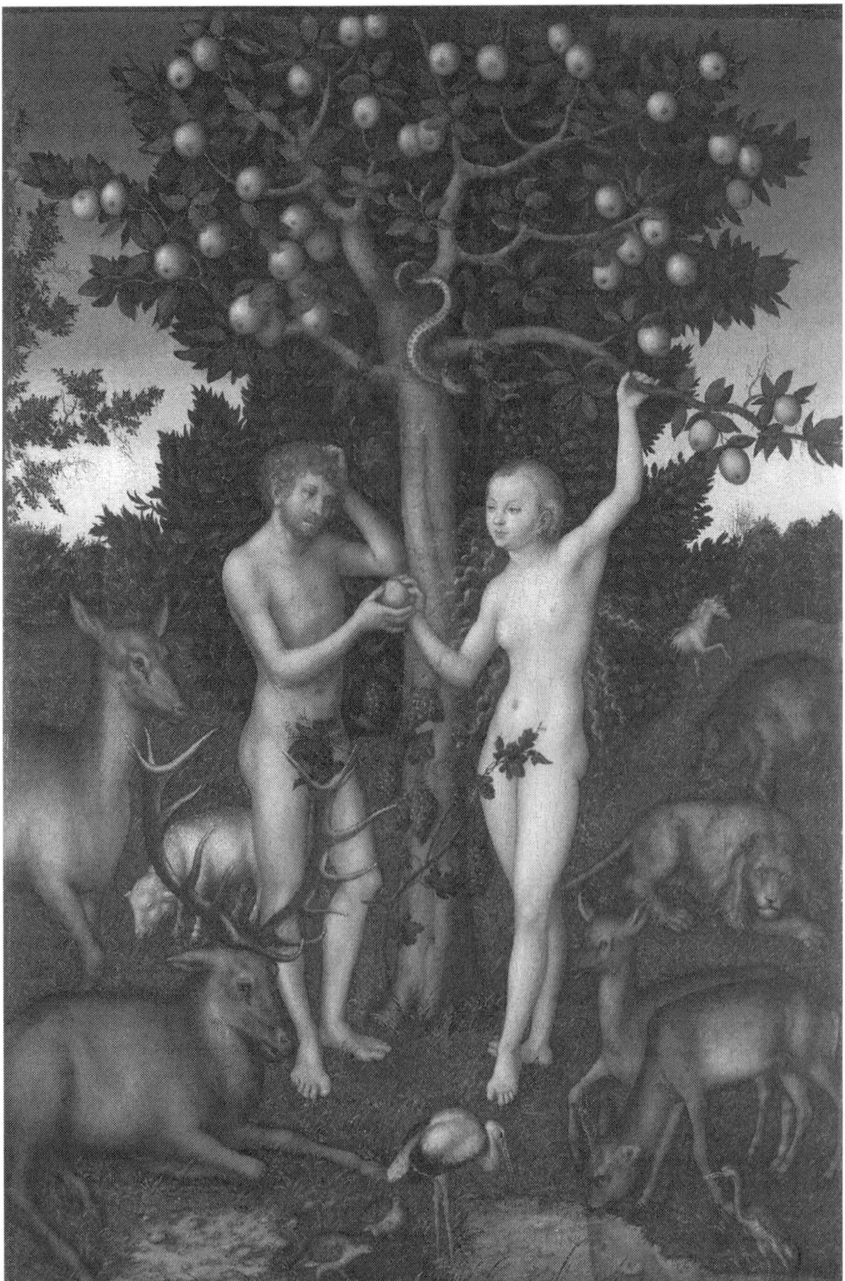

Adam and Eve, by Lucas Cranach the Elder

CONTENTS

This Book Is Not a Game

Every day of the week, many of us take a pill, it might be an antibiotic, a pill for skin or heart problems or an antidepressant. This story about ghost-writing and the hiding of clinical trial data, especially the data on what can go wrong on a pill, applies to every pill you might take.

But no-one tells you that you run these risks, and they don't tell the doctor prescribing a drug to you.

Instead, you and your doctors will find experts far and wide heaping scorn on the idea that anything could possibly go wrong on a prescription drug. These experts, bedecked though they might be with impressive credentials, rarely if ever have more expertise on working out if a drug causes an adverse event than you do. Few of them have any training in how to detect an adverse event.

This is a story about a chain of events in which someone like you—with no background in whether a drug could cause suicide or homicide—helped pierce the screen of fake expertise that companies hide behind. In this case the story hinges on a study in children of the selective serotonin reuptake inhibiting (SSRI) antidepressant paroxetine, branded as Paxil in the United States, Seroxat in the United Kingdom and a range or related names—Aropax, Deroxat—elsewhere.

It's a story that makes clear that motivation and common sense can be worth more than "expertise."

It is also a true story. Truth is stranger than fiction because fiction has to make sense.

In the interests of truth, it is sometimes necessary to leave holes in a story. In March 2004, at the height of concerns that what were then new wonder antidepressants might cause children to commit suicide, it looked as if the U.S. Food and Drug Administration (FDA) was going to claim there was no problem. However, Michelle Anderson from the office of Senator Chuck Grassley (R-Iowa) called a senior FDA honcho and immediately after her call, FDA gave the press an hour's notice of a briefing at which they effectively put a Black Box Warning on antidepressants.

What was said during that call? Was it a threat to expose the private peccadillos of the boss of FDA? The peccadillos of others are in here and how they play into this story, but we don't know what Andersen said.

After Black Box Warnings stained the SSRI antidepressants, Lady Macbeth like, senior FDA figures, working closely with trusted experts, spent over a decade trying to wash the stain away, in a manner that suggests the apparatus you think is there to look after you has no interest in truth, and many of those involved would prefer to see you dead than admit they got something wrong.

This is a true story about lies. In the case of suicide or homicide on SSRIs, the lie that fooled many for two decades was that concerns about antidepressants stemmed from pressure by the Church of Scientology. This lie was invented by or for Eli Lilly, the makers of Prozac. The lie was more potent than the Prozac it was invented to defend—a wonderful symbol of the fact that by the 1990s what were once pharmaceutical companies had become marketing companies—better at producing fictions than the medicines we desperately need.

Close to the entire medical literature you and your doctor rely on is now a lie in a different sense. It's a shame to reveal the denouement of a book before you get to the last page but here it is—if you think clinical trials should reveal truth in a way fiction doesn't you've lost touch with what is happening. The clinical trials at the heart of the evidence supposed to keep us safe are fictions. Company abilities to get away with this depend on being able to keep trial data filed away in places as inaccessible as the resting place of the Lost Ark.

This book's website comes with the only set of company Clinical Trial data that you, your doctor or others can access—not an absolutely complete set but enough for anyone to join us in the hunt for clues as to the best version of Study 329 and to a version of the story in this book with the least holes.

Nothing you will read here is juiced up. No scenes have been invented to make the story flow. This book is not a game.

Note: Interviews, references, videos, and transcripts cited in this book are available on Study329.org. See endnotes for details.

CHAPTER 1

Flying to Philadelphia

Shelley Jofre was 32 when she got on a plane to Philadelphia in May 2002. People teased her about looking even younger. She is short and slight. She's from Glasgow so her accent is distinctive even within the UK.

She joined the British Broadcasting Corporation's (BBC) flagship investigative program *Panorama* from BBC Scotland in 2000. One of her earliest programs was tackling the emerging use of stimulants for ADHD which was just starting in Britain. She picked David Healy as a possible interviewee. He was difficult to pin down. The only option seemed to be to get him while transiting through Manchester Airport when she was heading in the opposite direction. She ambushed him—and then discarded the interview.

Philadelphia was hosting the American Psychiatric Association's 2002 annual jamboree. There were close to 20,000 delegates. Jofre was travelling with her producer Ed Harriman, a suave, articulate American, who had persuaded the broadcaster to take on the practices of the pharmaceutical industry, now that GlaxoSmithKline (GSK) had become the world's largest pharmaceutical company and was based only a few miles away from BBC headquarters. He had an ace angle on a story about GSK's paroxetine—one of the best-selling drugs in the world.

After Jofre got on the flight, Harriman handed her an article by Martin Keller, Neal Ryan and others, referred to then as Keller et al or the Keller paper and later called Study 329. It was published in July 2001 in the *Journal of the American Academy of Child and Adolescent Psychopharmacology—JAACAP* to insiders. The leading journal in the field as it turned out.

Study 329 is a randomized clinical trial (RCT) of GSK's paroxetine, branded as Paxil in America, Seroxat in Britain, Deroxat in parts of Europe and Aropax in Australia. The trial involved depressed children recruited from centres in America and Canada. Harriman's angle was that he was pretty sure the children were being recruited from poor and deprived neighbourhoods and were likely to be mostly black. The mission—to document what was going on. Study 329 was one of the first major RCTs done with children. Harriman was sure it offered an opening on an unsavoury reality.

The flight from London was 8 hours. Time to read the article several times. There isn't much in it about the treatment centres. The article confidently claims Paxil is safe and effective—in its abstract, discussion and conclusion. But it also describes some of the children as becoming emotionally labile. Before they landed, Jofre told Harriman she was not clear this drug worked very well and wondered if it caused problems. This is not the story he said.

After landing, when interviewing American child psychiatrists attending APA, Harriman insisted Jofre stick to his script. But the questions he had given her got nowhere. Everyone looked puzzled at any hints the testing was happening in centres of deprivation.

Jofre called Healy from the meeting, asking if he'd read the article. No, he said. Do you know anything about where the testing happened? No. What does emotional lability mean? No idea.

One more interview left. With Neal Ryan, the second author on 329 and as it turned out the person who drew up the protocol for the study. At the best of times, Ryan looks uncomfortable but faced with questions about the treatment centres he looked very comfortable. Jofre ran out of questions early with some time left on the tape so she asked him about emotional lability. All of a sudden, Ryan looked intensely uncomfortable and she knew she was on to something but there wasn't time to find out what and Ryan wasn't hanging about.

As Neal Ryan retreated from the interview room, everyone's future changed. Ed Harriman didn't know it. He was right about a great deal, as it later turned out. GSK were running another trial, Study 377, which fit his bill. But he was not right about Study 329. He got dropped by *Panorama* who decided to follow Jofre's lead.

What came to light about Study 329 applies to every single drug anyone of any age takes for any medical condition. What came to light should shape the attitude everyone takes to every single academic article published in any area of medicine—it's bogus or semi-bogus until proven otherwise. Peer review is useless. Approval of a drug by a regulator means nothing. The greater the prestige of a medical journal the more it has invested in what drug companies want.

A few days later Jofre found that the April 2002 edition of *JAACAP* carried letters by Alex Weintrob from New York and Mitch Parsons from Edmonton about Study 329, mentioning their concerns about children becoming suicidal on SSRIs. A confident response from Keller and Ryan about the merits of controlled trials compared to anecdotes—the plural of anecdotes is not data—seemed like, for most people, it would deal a knockout blow to these anecdotes.

But Jofre was an anecdote person, as everyone who has anything go wrong on a drug necessarily is, and these letters fit her hunch.

Four years later at an APA meeting in Toronto, she interviewed Martin Keller. This time she came armed. She had been working with George W Murgatroyd III, Skip to everyone who knows him. Skip is a lawyer who shares a gift with her—that of being able to vanish into the background.

It worked when Skip deposed Marty Keller the apparent author of Study 329 under oath and then when he deposed the real author of the study, whose name features nowhere.

It worked in Toronto when Jofre interviewed Keller, a tall, slim, handsome and confident man, whose photographs don't do him justice. He is as comfortable in his body as Ryan is uncomfortable. He didn't smell danger when Jofre approached him for a quick question after his lecture. This was not a formal interview setting. Who could think such a young-looking girl could pose a threat? Not a camera or tape recorder in sight.

JOFRE: *What about suicide attempts on Paxil?*

KELLER: *None of these attempts led to suicide and very few of them led to hospitalization. The thing is, you have to consider what are the alternatives? Right?*

JOFRE: *So some of the unpublished studies showed that placebo actually seemed to have more of an effect?*

KELLER: *Come on, you know better than that.*

And reaching down from a height he stroked Shelley Jofre under the chin. A touch that Hans Christian Andersen missed.

CHAPTER 2

Girl on a Plane

At this point, you can try the Girl-on-a-Plane test. The full Keller paper is on Study 329.org in its original formatting, along with the reviews of the original paper and all letters linked to it.

If you have never read an academic paper before, don't be put off. Shelley Jofre flying to Philadelphia had read few papers. In her case, this seems to have been an advantage, rather than a drawback.

Reading the original doesn't mean understanding every word. Most academics and doctors skip the methods section unless they are very bored. They might look at the results tables, but details like these often anesthetise rather than illuminate, and they are there in part for that purpose. Besides none of the academics who should have spotted the problems in the methods or results sections did so. Some of the self-proclaimed world's leading experts on clinical trials apparently still can't see the problems. You are more likely to spot the problems if your job doesn't depend on not seeing them.

Essentially doctors read the abstract, which we reproduce in full below. Some of them then might read the introduction before glazing over and skipping to the discussion.

We summarize the introduction, methods, results and discussion for you below, which you can read in lieu of reading the paper, or you can read both and see what you think of our summary.

After the paper, or the summary, there is fork in the road. Chapters three to five give a background for depression, antidepressants, suicide and treatment, and where the selective serotonin reuptake inhibitor (SSRI) group of drugs come from. These chapters are not reference heavy. There are a few linked documents and interviews with the people who actually made the discoveries, available on Study329.org, which may leave some figuring that what they thought was rocket science is more like the making and flying of paper airplanes.

Or you can skip to Chapter Six, which will land you in Philadelphia with Shelley Jofre. She knew less about serotonin, antidepressants and suicide when she arrived there than any readers who travel via Chapters Three to Five. You can double back to the chapters on depression and serotonin at any point, if you need to make sure the bizarre world that started opening up in Philly in 2002 is for real or not.

When you get to Chapter Eleven, there is *The Girl with a Headache Test*. At this point your option is to read the Le Noury et al paper, or our summary of it, or both.

Efficacy of Paroxetine in the Treatment of Adolescent Major Depression: A Randomized, Controlled Trial

MARTIN B. KELLER, M.D., NEAL D. RYAN, M.D., MICHAEL STROBER, PH.D., RACHEL G. KLEIN, PH.D., STAN P. KUTCHER, M.D., BORIS BIRMAHER, M.D., OWEN R. HAGINO, M.D., HAROLD KOPLEWICZ, M.D., GABRIELLE A. CARLSON, M.D., GREGORY N. CLARKE, PH.D., GRAHAM J. EMSLIE, M.D., DAVID FEINBERG, M.D., BARBARA GELLER, M.D., VIVEK KUSUMAKAR, M.D., GEORGE PAPATHEODOROU, M.D., WILLIAM H. SACK, M.D., MICHAEL SWEENEY, PH.D., KAREN DINEEN WAGNER, M.D., PH.D., ELIZABETH B. WELLER, M.D., NANCY C. WINTERS, M.D., ROSEMARY OAKES, M.S., AND JAMES P. MCCAFFERTY, B.S.

ABSTRACT

Objective: To compare paroxetine with placebo and imipramine with placebo for the treatment of adolescent depression. **Method:** After a 7- to 14-day screening period, 275 adolescents with major depression began 8 weeks of double-blind paroxetine (20–40 mg), imipramine (gradual upward titration to 200–300 mg), or placebo. The two primary outcome measures were endpoint response (Hamilton Rating Scale for Depression [HAM-D] score ≤8 or ≥50% reduction in baseline HAM-D) and change from baseline HAM-D score. Other depression-related variables were (1) HAM-D depressed mood item; (2) depression item of the Schedule for Affective Disorders and Schizophrenia for Adolescents-Lifetime version (K-SADS-L); (3) Clinical Global Impression (CGI) improvement scores of 1 or 2; (4) nine-item depression subscale of K-SADS-L; and (5) mean CGI improvement scores. **Results:** Paroxetine demonstrated significantly greater improvement compared with placebo in HAM-D total score ≤8, HAM-D depressed mood item, K-SADS-L depressed mood item, and CGI score of 1 or 2. The response to imipramine was not significantly different from placebo for any measure. Neither paroxetine nor imipramine differed significantly from placebo on parent- or self-rating measures. Withdrawal rates for adverse effects were 9.7% and 6.9% for paroxetine and placebo, respectively. Of 31.5% of subjects stopping imipramine therapy because of adverse effects, nearly one third did so because of adverse cardiovascular effects. **Conclusions:** Paroxetine is generally well tolerated and effective for major depression in adolescents. J. Am. Acad. Child Adolesc. Psychiatry, 2001, 40(7):762–772. **Key Words:** paroxetine, imipramine, major depression, adolescent.

This study was supported by a grant from GlaxoSmithKline, Collegeville, PA. Editorial assistance was provided by Sally K. Laden, M.S.

Reprint requests to Dr. Keller, Department of Psychiatry and Human Behavior, Brown University School of Medicine, 345 Blackstone Blvd., Providence, RI 02906.

INTRODUCTION

Until recently we didn't think children became depressed, but we have now discovered, thanks primarily to the work of Martin Keller, that one in six adolescents is significantly depressed with an illness indistinguishable from major depressive disorder in adults. This often runs a prolonged and recurrent course and if left untreated will mean that these adolescents are at risk of career failure, marital breakdown, alcoholism, substance abuse, or suicide.

Older antidepressants like imipramine came with a heavy burden of side effects for this age group. There have been a number of studies of these older drugs in this age group, none of which have been shown to work. But until now there have been no proper RCTs. It has only been with the advent of the new SSRI antidepressants that the first proper studies have been undertaken. One of these studies produced a positive result for Prozac. This is a bigger and more ambitious study, comparing paroxetine, imipramine, and placebo.

METHODS

This was an 8-week RCT comparing paroxetine with a placebo and imipramine in adolescents with major depression, conducted at 12 North American centres. A total of 275 subjects were involved. The trial was conducted according to the highest standards, and all children and their parent(s) gave consent. GSK funded the study. Each author had access to the data and signed off on the manuscript.

The subjects were aged 12 through 18 years and met criteria for major depression. The diagnosis was made using a standard interview adapted for children, and all children had a total score of at least 12 on the 17-item Hamilton Rating Scale for Depression (HAM-D).

We excluded all children who had any other disorder or who were suicidal or who had any medical condition for which the use of an antidepressant was contraindicated, as well as children who had had any psychotropic drug use within the previous six months or exposure to investigational drug use within 30 days of study entry. We also excluded all girls who were pregnant or breast-feeding, or who were sexually active but not using reliable contraception.

After screening for 1–2 weeks, subjects who were still depressed entered the study and were randomly given paroxetine, imipramine, or a placebo for 8 weeks, with all pills made up to be indistinguishable one from the other. Subjects taking paroxetine began at 20 mg and after Week 4 could increase to 30 mg or 40 mg if clinically indicated. Imipramine began at 50 mg and was increased by 50 mg per week to 200 mg during Week 4. It could then be increased to 250 mg or 300 mg if clinically necessary.

Subjects who completed the study were offered the option of continuing blinded treatment at the same dose for 6 additional months. If subjects withdrew from the study prematurely for any reason, the dose of medication was gradually tapered over a 7- to 17-day period.

We used standard rating scales at weekly intervals to determine whether the drug was working. We defined a response to treatment as a HAM-D score of 8 or less and a 50% reduction in baseline HAM-D score at the end of treatment; and (2) change from baseline in HAM-D total score. In addition we had a number of other measures of effectiveness, and we used a number of other more general scales.

Adverse events, heart rate, blood pressure, and body weight were determined weekly, keeping a particular eye on the cardiovascular changes linked to imipramine in this dose.

We used absolutely standard statistical tests for analysing the data.

RESULTS

Most of the children had been depressed for a year or more. Many of them were severely depressed. One third were male, two thirds female. The average age was 15, and 77% were white.

By the end of the study on most of the measures, paroxetine was statistically better than placebo, whereas there was no difference between imipramine and placebo. Overall, 63% of paroxetine children, 50% of imipramine children, and 46% of placebo children showed a response.

FIGURE: MEAN CHANGE IN HAM-D

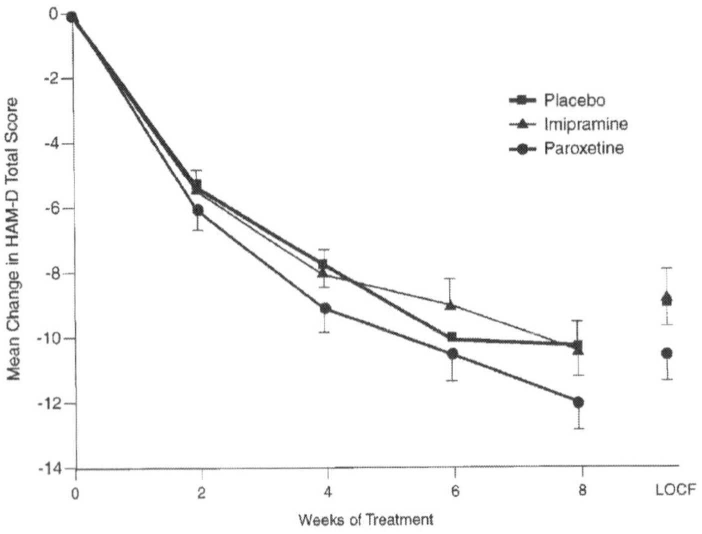

Among children taking a placebo, 24% dropped out, 7% for adverse events. Among children taking paroxetine, 28% dropped out, 10% for adverse events. Among children taking imipramine, 40% dropped out, 32% for adverse events, mainly cardiovascular events.

Paroxetine was well tolerated, and most adverse effects were not serious. The most common problems were headache, nausea, dizziness, dry mouth, and somnolence. These occurred at rates that were similar to rates in the placebo group with the exception of somnolence, which occurred at rates of 17% for paroxetine and 3% for placebo. Dizziness, dry mouth, headache, nausea, and tachycardia were most commonly reported during imipramine treatment. Tremor occurred in 11% of paroxetine, 15% of imipramine, and 2% of placebo subjects. There were no clinically significant changes in weight.

TABLE

Adverse Effects Occurring in Paroxetine, Imipramine, and Placebo Subjects

Adverse Effect	Paroxetine (n = 93)		Imipramine (n = 95)		Placebo (n = 87)	
Nervous system						
Dizziness	22	(23.7)	45	(47.4)	16	(18.4)
Emotional lability	6	(6.5)	3	(3.2)	1	(1.1)
Hostility	7	(7.5)	3	(3.2)	0	(0)
Insomnia	14	(15.1)	13	(13.7)	4	(4.6)
Nervousness	8	(8.6)	6	(6.3)	5	(5.7)
Somnolence	16	(17.2)	13	(13.7)	3	(3.4)
Tremor	10	(10.8)	14	(14.7)	2	(2.3)
Headache	32	(34.4)	38	(40.0)	34	(39.1)
Trauma	2	(2.2)	3	(3.2)	6	(6.9)

Serious adverse effects occurred in 11 paroxetine children, 5 imipramine children, and 2 placebo children. The serious paroxetine events consisted of headache during discontinuation (one patient) and psychiatric events in 10 patients: worsening depression in 2; emotional lability (e.g., suicidal ideation/

gestures) in 5; conduct problems or hostility in 2; and euphoria in 1. Seven patients were hospitalized: 2 with worsening depression, 2 with emotional lability, 2 with conduct problems, and 1 with euphoria. Of the 11 patients, only headache was considered by the treating investigator to be caused by paroxetine.

The 5 serious adverse effects in the imipramine group consisted of maculopapular rash in 1 patient, breathlessness/ chest pain in 1, hostility in 1, emotional lability in 1, and visual hallucinations/abnormal dreams in 1. The rash and hallucinations were thought to be caused by imipramine. All 5 patients were withdrawn from the study, and the patients with hostility or emotional lability were hospitalized.

In the placebo group, there was emotional lability in 1 and worsening depression in 1. The emotional lability was considered to be caused by placebo, and the patient was withdrawn from the study.

DISCUSSION

This is the first study to compare an SSRI like paroxetine with one of the older antidepressants and a placebo. It showed that paroxetine works, which was in line with our clinical impressions of giving SSRIs to adolescents. Because no studies have shown that older antidepressants work and their side effects are so severe, they are unlikely to be used much in future.

The adverse-effect profile of paroxetine for adolescents was similar to that found in depressed adults. Serious adverse effects were reported with paroxetine (11 patients), imipramine (5), and placebo (2). Because these serious adverse effects were judged by the investigator to be related to treatment in only 4 patients (paroxetine 1; imipramine 2; placebo 1), we cannot be certain treatment caused them. There were no cardiovascular effects with paroxetine, but these were severe for imipramine.

There was a high placebo response rate in this study, which is not unusual. It may have been caused partly by the weekly visits. We don't fully understand this.

Major depression in adolescents is increasingly recognized. Tricyclic antidepressants are not recommended for use in this age group. Despite some methodological limitations, resulting in a high placebo response rate, our study demonstrates that treatment with paroxetine produces responses. The SSRIs are the treatment of choice in this age group because they are the only agents that have been shown to work; they are safer than other antidepressants, particularly in overdose, and they can be given once a day. In actual clinical practice, children may do even better than they did here.

CONCLUSION

The findings of this study show paroxetine is effective and safe for adolescents who are depressed. We need more studies to work out the best dose and how long to continue treatment.

REFERENCES

See references and the complete study as published in July 2001 in the *Journal of the American Association for Child and Adolescent Psychiatry,* (*JAACAP*) on www.study329.org

CHAPTER 3

Depression: An Illness is Born

Before 1985, depression was a rare disorder—several thousand times less common than it is now thought to be. Few psychiatrists and even fewer doctors would have diagnosed it in children. When we were nervous or had nervous breakdowns, we were seen as suffering from anxiety, or, after the publication of DSM III in 1980, we had one of the anxiety disorders. "Nerves" came with an increased heart rate, butterflies in the stomach or other gastrointestinal complaints, headaches, sweating, and breathlessness. Freud and psychoanalysis did a great deal to portray nerves as anxiety and to entrench talking therapies as the necessary approach to get to the root of what was bothering us[1].

The world wars brought home the idea that extreme environmental stress could produce "nervous breakdowns." For broken soldiers sedation was often the answer. Opiates or alcohol were the sedatives of choice in the nineteenth century, before various bromides and barbiturates replaced them. In the 1930s, stimulants like dexamphetamine appeared, followed by combinations of stimulants and sedatives such as Dexamyl—a combination of dexamphetamine and amylobarbitone.

Then in a few short years around World War II, medicine was transformed by a pharmacological revolution that began with the antibiotics and antihistamines.

In the 1950s, two groups of drugs, the major and minor tranquilizers, appeared. Chlorpromazine—branded as Thorazine in the United States and Largactil in Europe—was the first of the major tranquilizers. It has been described as one of the ten most important discoveries in medicine. Initially called a tranquilizer or neuroleptic, it was the precursor to all later antipsychotics and antidepressants.

But when it came to North America, it had to share the stage with meprobamate, which launched under the brand name Miltown looked like the bigger drug. Meprobamate was discovered by Frank Berger, who immigrated to the United States from Czechoslovakia before the war. Berger was working in the laboratories of Carter Wallace on muscle relaxants when he discovered that meprobamate calmed laboratory animals without unduly sedating them. Since muscular tension was a feature of anxiety, he reasoned that muscular relaxation without sedation might be good for anxiety states. Given that his new drug was less sedative than older ones, Berger adopted a term that had been recently coined—Miltown would be a tranquilizer.

Miltown looked to be the ideal answer for everyday anxiety. It produced a pleasant, relaxed feeling, which "liberated" people from their nerves, encouraging them to do things they would not have done otherwise. It left many people feeling better than well. A Miltown craze spread through newspapers, radio and the emerging medium of television[2].

A few years later it was gone, supplanted by even more perfect tranquilizers. Librium and Valium emerged in the early 1960s. These benzodiazepine drugs were as effective as Miltown with even less sedation. Hoffman La Roche marketed them brilliantly, "helping" doctors to realize that a significant proportion of the physical complaints appearing in their offices might be manifestations of anxiety. What drove ulcers if not anxiety? No one knew what caused hypertension, but it sounded as though these patients were bottling up their anxiety. Patients with asthma or other breathing conditions were often anxious, as were patients with headaches. In all of these conditions it became common to prescribe a tranquilizer along with whatever else the patient was taking. Physicians gave Valium to college students facing the stresses of their new environment. Housewives were prescribed Valium to cope with the stresses of new suburban lifestyles. Busy executives were taking it too. By 1970 Valium was the best-selling drug in the world.

Critics questioned the wisdom of mass tranquilization. Would these drugs dull the natural competitiveness people need in a hard world? Would nations become less fit for survival if these drugs were overused? Problems coping at college surely were not medical disorders. The student revolutionaries of the late 1960s argued it was the political system that was confusing and disorienting people, and that the appropriate therapeutic intervention was not to treat individuals but to change the system. Women seeking liberation claimed they were being doped into submission.

The benzodiazepine bandwagon shuddered to a halt in the 1980s. But the undoing of the "benzos" came not because we turned against mass prescribing to mask social ills. It came when the possibility was raised in the late 1970s that these drugs that had been so relied upon might lead to dependence. The spectre of dependence provoked a crisis that in turn helped create health news. Before 1980, it was unusual to see health coverage in major newspapers. Stories about benzodiazepines now began to appear regularly, helping create the phenomenon of a regular health page in newspapers. Talk shows on which individuals discuss their problems, like *Donahue* and *Oprah* in the United States and *That's Life* in England, fostered these developments. Health was a natural subject for these shows; the coverage they provided led to coalitions of patients campaigning on matters like benzodiazepine dependence[3].

The experts pushed back against the idea benzodiazepines were addictive. They pointed out that animal tests for abuse liability showed benzodiazepines were very different from heroin, cocaine and other drugs prone to abuse. Addicts might use benzos, but they had little street value. These were good drugs, and most patients were able to discontinue benzodiazepines without difficulty.

But these establishment views sank beneath a rising tide of discontent. Until then, addicts had been socially shunned as the perpetrators of their own downfall. But benzodiazepine "addicts" were seen as victims of a medico-pharmaceutical establishment. Doctors and drug companies became the villains.[4] The benzodiazepines rapidly passed from being seen as remarkably safe medicines to being seen as one of the greatest dangers to modern society.

But, it was not the critics who brought the benzos down. It was other pharmaceutical companies. Another group of drugs active on the serotonin system was in clinical trials, of which buspirone (Buspar) was later the best known. Mead-Johnson in America and Bristol-Myers Squib in Britain were prepared to highlight the problems of the benzodiazepines as part of a campaign to market buspirone as the first non-dependence producing anxiolytic.

This is the usual way the problems of drugs come to light. It's not through doctors or the media. It's when companies have a different set of on-patent drugs to market, and they decide to highlight the problems of previous drugs that have gone off-patent. This message is progress incarnate.

In this case, the tactic had a mixed result—Buspar flopped. But the benzodiazepine crisis had educated physicians to expect that any drug that treated anxiety would in due course be found to cause dependence. This wasn't a gentle education—specialists speaking on company platforms told generalists in the audience that they would be sued if they prescribed benzodiazepines. The education was so effective that it became impossible to persuade physicians or patients that there could be a non-dependence-producing tranquilizer. Rebranding these new drugs as anxiolytics didn't do it. The tranquilizer era was over, and the antidepressant era was about to start.

The challenge for companies was to translate cases of Valium into cases of Prozac. They did such a good job that to this day among the wider public Valium is seen as a darker drug than Prozac or Paxil or Zoloft. But if forced to take a benzodiazepine or an SSRI for a year, most people working in mental health, if given a choice, would opt for the benzodiazepine.

The antidepressant era

Conventionally, the antidepressant story starts in 1957 with the twin discoveries of Geigy's tricyclic antidepressant, imipramine, by Roland Kuhn, and of Roche's monoamine oxidase inhibitor (MAOI), iproniazid, by Nathan Kline. Neither Geigy nor Roche had much interest in an antidepressant—the market was too small.

When Merck launched another antidepressant, amitriptyline, in 1961, unlike Geigy and Roche, they decided to market depression as well as amitriptyline. That year, Frank Ayd from Baltimore had published a book titled *Recognizing the Depressed Patient.* Merck commissioned 50,000 copies and distributed it to physicians and psychiatrists. Amitriptyline quickly became the best-selling of this group of drugs, later called the tricyclic antidepressants (TCAs or tricyclics) because of their three-ringed molecular structure. Despite Merck's efforts, however, antidepressants remained poor cousins of the tranquilizers.[5]

During the 1960s and 1970s, many senior psychiatrists argued that a significant number of patients diagnosed as anxious were in fact depressed, and further, that the appropriate treatment for them was an antidepressant rather than a tranquilizer. This vision led Paul Kielholz, a professor of psychiatry in Geigy's hometown of Basel, Switzerland, to set up the first meeting of the Committee for the Prevention and Treatment of Depression in 1972.[6]

Meanwhile, in 1966, Michael Shepherd in London published the first study examining the nervous problems that family doctors were seeing—patients psychiatrists never saw. Shepherd concluded that many of these problems could be viewed as depression. This and later studies in the 1980s found more than enough depression to attract the interest of companies then developing a new group of drugs acting on the serotonin system[7].

Another development that helped to open up a depression market came with the creation of the third edition of the American Psychiatric Association's *Diagnostic and Statistical Manual of Mental Disorders—DSM-III.* Following the introduction of the new psychotropic drugs in the 1950s, there was a split in American psychiatry between analysts who saw psychotherapy as the only appropriate treatment and physicians who began using the new antipsychotics and antidepressants. This split was aggravated in the late 1960s by an antipsychiatry movement, which questioned the legitimacy of all psychiatric diagnoses and practices. These conflicts led in 1980 to the introduction of operational criteria for psychiatric disorders in a revised diagnostic manual, *DSM-III*.

In *DSM-III*, anxiety was broken down into a number of apparently different disorders—social phobia, generalized anxiety disorder, panic disorder, post-traumatic stress disorder and obsessive-compulsive disorder. This is exactly what companies seeking to develop an anxiety market wanted. In contrast, depressive disorders were collapsed into one large category—major depressive disorder.

Segmentation of a market is usually what pharmaceutical companies want but in this case lumping all types of depression together turned out to be the jackpot move. It enabled the SSRIs, which have very weak effects on any depression, to be marketed as working for major depressive disorder and therefore seeming potent and even more important to be marketed for primary care nerves.

DSM III's new formulations came on stream just as Kielholz's Committee for the Prevention and Treatment of Depression laid the foundation for campaigns such as *Depression Awareness, Recognition, and Treatment (DART)* in the United States and *Defeat Depression* in the United Kingdom. As these campaigns took shape, Eli Lilly decided to put a major effort into promoting Prozac for depression. In the case of DART, Lilly's money supported eight million copies of a brochure titled *Depression: What You Need to Know* and 200,000 posters. As Lew Judd, the Director of the National Institute of Mental Health (NIMH), put it in 1987, "By making these materials on depressive illness available, accessible in physicians' offices all over the country, important information is effectively reaching the public in settings which encourage questions, discussion, treatment, or referral."

Campaigns like this can do great good—or they can be self-serving. In the early 1990s, surveys by the *Defeat Depression* Campaign in Britain found that most people thought depression was not the kind of condition that should be treated with pills. But the 1980s saw a dramatic increase in articles about depression in both medical journals and general readership magazines.

Both academic and lay media were reporting benzodiazepine horror stories, in contrast to the feel-good stories of previous years. There was scope for stories about a new feel-good drug. And so, the kinds of stories that clinicians like Nathan Kline and Paul Kielholz had been trying to cultivate for years, previously choked of light by the canopy of overhanging tranquilizer publicity, were given a chance to grow.

The depression campaigns told physicians and healthcare funders that untreated depression caused a huge economic burden. The campaigns were so successful that within a decade no one questioned claims that depression was one of the greatest single health burdens on humanity. But no one seemed to require proof that treatments designed to make a difference actually did produce benefits. There is plenty of evidence that antidepressants can be shown to do something in the short term but almost no evidence that patients are better off in the long run. Something must surely be going wrong if the frequency of depression has apparently jumped a thousand-fold since the introduction of the antidepressants.

A series of educational campaigns to show physicians how many cases of depression they were missing was designed to shame them into detecting and treating depression. This new emphasis now causes many people to end up being diagnosed with depression who do not regard themselves as being depressed or in need of treatment. In individual cases this heightening of clinician sensitivity to depression may have saved lives, but there is no evidence that mass detection and treatment has lowered national suicide or disability rates.

The antidepressant story has a further important twist. In the early 1980s, the conventional wisdom was that—unlike tranquilizers, which were feel-good agents that delivered a relatively immediate payoff—antidepressants took several weeks to work. Prescribers were educated to tell patients that they could even expect to feel worse for some weeks before they began to feel better. This strategy gave the message that these were not quick-fix pills, but rather serious medications that would correct the problem.

But this same educational information sets up a trap. For many doctors the idea that SSRI antidepressants might lead to suicide or other problems during the early period "before the pills begin working" seemed a contradiction in terms.

Patients faced with a doctor who doesn't believe a treatment can be causing problems in the first few weeks can be trapped by the relationship with their doctor. Where they would probably discontinue an over-the-counter medication if it did not seem to suit them, regard for their doctor traps them into continuing treatment especially when the doctor tells them the treatment takes more time to work. Continuing with a treatment that might kill them.

Just as the new serotonergic drugs had to kill off the benzodiazepines and did so by playing the addiction and dependence card, they also had to clear out the older tricyclic antidepressants. In this case, the weapon was safety in overdose. Unlike the TCAs, which can be dangerous in overdose, an SSRI it was claimed couldn't be used to commit suicide.

The older tricyclics were effective drugs that in many cases brought about responses in patients with melancholic or even psychotic depression. But these were rare disorders, and never present in children. There is an assumption that patients with melancholia have something biologically wrong with them—they cannot sleep, they become almost parkinsonian in their movements and thinking, they stop eating and may die if not force-fed, and they are at high risk of suicide. But no-one knows what the biological problem is.

Serotonin and depression

For many people a belief that serotonin is low in depression is one of the key factors that make it reasonable to take an antidepressant. Even for those who are against drugs for nervous problems, taking something that restores you to normal sounds almost like an ethical duty.

The presence in the brain of serotonin was first reported in 1954.[8] This quickly led to the hypothesis that this monoamine neurotransmitter might play some role in nervous problems. One way to investigate this possibility was to look at the levels of the main breakdown products of serotonin (5HIAA) in the cerebrospinal fluid that bathes the brain. In 1960, George Ashcroft, working in Edinburgh, found that cerebrospinal 5HIAA levels in depressives appeared to be low. He put forward the first theory that serotonin might be low in depression. The following year, Ashcroft and others reported that it might be high in people with autism. The autism claim still holds water, but by the end of the 1960s even Ashcroft had abandoned the link between serotonin and depression[9].

While Europe was convinced that serotonin was a key neurotransmitter, Americans were certain norepinephrine was more important. Julius Axelrod, working at the National Institutes of Health (NIH), had discovered an uptake mechanism for norepinephrine in 1961 that tricyclic antidepressants like imipramine blocked[10]. Axelrod dismissed serotonin as just "a remnant of our marine past."

In 1965, Joseph Schildkraut at the National Institute of Mental Health published the key article of the new biological psychiatry, its *Interpretation of Dreams*, the "Catecholamine Hypothesis of Depression."[11] In it, Schildkraut put forward the idea that norepinephrine levels were lowered in depression and antidepressants increased the levels. Whatever the scientific basis for this claim, it represented a new language that both physicians and patients could understand. Freudian talk of sexual complexes yielded to a new patter: "You have a chemical imbalance; these pills will restore your brain to normal." Magazines from *Time* and *Newsweek* to *The New Republic* and *The National Enquirer* could embrace this idea, which became crucial to the later success of Prozac. This key myth still flourishes in popular consciousness more than 50 years later.

By the mid-1970s, it was clear there was nothing wrong with serotonin or norepinephrine levels in depression. Indeed, no abnormality of serotonin in depression has ever been demonstrated. When the SSRIs launched in the 1990s, there was no correlation between how potent a serotonin reuptake inhibitor any of these drugs were and how good an antidepressant they were. No one even knew if SSRIs raised or lowered serotonin levels. They still don't know. The evidence suggests that SSRIs lower serotonin in some patients and that this may link to suicidality and impulsiveness.

In the 1990s, when the SSRIs were being marketed, no academic could state publicly that serotonin was low in people with depression. So the role of persuading people to restore their serotonin levels to "normal" fell to patient representatives and patient groups—heavily sponsored by pharmaceutical companies. The lowered serotonin story took root in the public domain. The public's concept of serotonin was like Freud's notion of libido—vague, and incapable of testing. It was the perfect piece of biobabble to replace the previously dominant psychobabble. If researchers used this language, it was in the form of a symbol referring to some physiological abnormality that most still presumed would be found to underpin melancholia—although not necessarily primary care "depression."

The myth co-opted the complementary health market as well. Alternative health books routinely encourage people to eat foods or engage in activities that will enhance their serotonin levels. In so doing, these books, whose authors are competing with psychiatry, confirm the validity of using an antidepressant. The myth also co-opts psychologists and others, who for instance attempt to explain the evolutionary significance of depression in terms of the function of the serotonin system. Journals and publishers accept books and articles like these because they believe the role of lowering serotonin in relation to depression is an established fact. And in so doing, all these people, who are mostly hostile to the pharmaceutical industry, help sell antidepressants.

Above all, the myth co-opted primary care doctors and patients. For doctors it provided an easy shorthand for communication with patients. For patients, the idea of correcting an abnormality has a moral force that can be expected to overcome their scruples about using a tranquilizer, especially when packaged in the appealing form that the distress they feel is not a weakness—it's an illness like diabetes.

At the same time as this triumph of "biological" language was taking place, the field abandoned another set of findings. By the mid-1970s, melancholia or severe mood disorder had been firmly linked to elevations of the stress hormone cortisol. The SSRIs however are ineffective in severe mood disorders where cortisol is raised. Real biology would have killed the SSRIs, but astonishingly research on cortisol in mood disorders was eclipsed instead.

Serotonin is not irrelevant. Neurotransmitters like serotonin and norepinephrine do vary among individuals, and there is likely some correlation between our transmitter profiles and our temperaments and personalities. Indeed, there is some research linking lowered serotonin metabolite levels with impulsivity leading to suicidality, aggression and alcoholism—and even evidence that SSRIs lower serotonin while leading to these problems.

These issues matter. In other areas of life, the products we use, from computers to microwaves, generally improve from one year to the next. This is not, however, the case for medicines where this year's treatments may achieve blockbuster sales despite being less effective and less safe than yesterday's models.

The emerging sciences of the brain offer enormous scope to deploy any amount of biobabble. There will be a growing need in years to come for us all to understand the language we hear. Unless some extraordinary change occurs, you should start by assuming that well over half of what you hear confidently put forward as known science is actually marketing junk. You might even be safe to treat all of it as junk and concentrate on making sure your doctor can actually see or hear what is happening to you.

CHAPTER 4

The Birth of the SSRIs

The origin of the Selective Serotonin Reuptake Inhibitors (SSRIs), also lies with Paul Kielholz after he became professor of psychiatry in Basel. Given the presence in Basel of the major Swiss chemical companies, Geigy, Ciba and Sandoz (all later to merge to become Novartis), Kielholz was well placed to become a leader in world psychopharmacology. Depression, which he saw as underrecognized and poorly treated, was his area of interest. More had to be done, he argued, than simply teach physicians to detect depression and put patients on treatment. Different antidepressants did quite different things, and it was important to select the right antidepressant for the individual patient.[12]

While the tricyclic molecular structures of the early antidepressants all looked very similar, Kielholz argued that some of them, such as desipramine, helped people by enhancing drive, while others, such as trimipramine, helped through a sedative action. Still others had some other effect on mood or emotions that he found difficult to characterize. Clomipramine, imipramine and amitriptyline appeared to have more of this mysterious effect than other tricyclic antidepressants.

This observation flew in the face of Schildkraut's catecholamine theory, which claimed that all antidepressants worked to inhibit norepinephrine reuptake. It took Arvid Carlsson, a new kind of player within psychopharmacology, to resolve the issue. Carlsson, a Swede, was one of the first neuroscientists. Trained in Steve Brodie's laboratory in the U.S. National Institutes of Health, he had a string of early research successes to his credit, including demonstrating the existence of neurotransmitter pathways in the brain. He had discovered dopamine and was among the first to suggest it might be abnormal in Parkinson's, work that later led to a Nobel Prize. As early as 1963, he had put forward the first evidence that led to the dopamine hypothesis of schizophrenia[13].

Carlsson saw a connection between the different effects Kielholz claimed and the effects of these drugs on neurotransmitter systems. The drugs Kielholz characterized as drive-enhancing had effects on the norepinephrine system, whereas clomipramine in particular had effects on both the serotonin and norepinephrine systems. This led Carlsson to suggest developing drugs that selectively inhibited serotonin reuptake with little effects on norepinephrine to see if a pure drug might tell us more about the nature of this mysterious other action, and also let us see what manipulating serotonin might do for depression.

Being able to detect an effect when a drug is acting on a brain system assumes there is no abnormality in that system. If there were an abnormality of the serotonin system, which SSRIs corrected, these drugs should be among the most potent antidepressants. But in fact they are among the weakest.

So, if Kielholz was right, the question is what do SSRIs tell us about this mysterious other action. All the evidence suggests it's a tranquilizing action—like Buspar. Such an action would explain why SSRIs are useful across a range of mixed anxiety and depressive states. But Buspar had shown drugs like this could not be marketed as a non-dependence producing tranquilizer even if tranquilizers were rebranded as anxiolytics.

Zelmid: the first SSRI

Working with Astra in Sweden, Carlsson manipulated an antihistamine, chlorpheniramine, and came up with zimelidine. This was patented as a selective serotonin reuptake inhibitor to be used for treating depression on April 28, 1971, three years before Prozac.

Zimelidine went into clinical trials to compare it with desipramine, a norepinephrine reuptake inhibitor. These were short trials in mild to moderate depression—not melancholia. The first results were presented in 1980, and zimelidine launched in Europe as Zelmid in 1982—six years before Prozac.

Zelmid was marketed heavily and widely prescribed in Europe. Astra had signed an agreement with Merck to market Zelmid in the United States. Merck was the largest pharmaceutical company in the world at the time and recognized as marketers par excellence. Had it launched Zelmid in the United States, Prozac would never have become a household name. But just as the data on Zelmid were delivered to the FDA in 1982, reports appeared linking it to Guillain-Barré Syndrome. This neurological disorder, which can kill by paralyzing respiratory muscles, led to Zelmid's removal from the market.

Astra was taking no chances, in part because it already had another SSRI, alaproclate, in development. But alaproclate was later found to cause liver problems in a strain of mice, and it too was dropped. Shortly after that, Astra introduced an innovative antipsychotic, remoxipride, which seemed to have fewer side effects than older antipsychotics but soon after its launch, it was reported to cause aplastic anemia in a small number of people, and it too was withdrawn.

In the face of these setbacks, Astra contemplated withdrawing from the research-based market to focus on over-the-counter medicines. It kept going only because it had the breakthrough anti-ulcer drug omeprazole, the first proton-pump inhibitor, which became one of the best-selling drugs on the market. Despite the revenues from omeprazole under the brand names Losec and Prilosec, Astra was forced to merge later in the decade with a newly branded British company—Zeneca Pharmaceuticals, formerly ICI.

Drug development stakes had become huge by 1990. A troublesome side effect early in the life of a new compound can lead to the demise of a company. But what if, rather than a side effect, the problem—for example, suicidality in the case of an antidepressant—could be portrayed as a feature of the disease being treated? If the alternative was going out of business, what would a company do?

During early clinical trials and post-launch studies, patients taking Zelmid had a greater number of suicide attempts than expected. No one knew what to make of this. Was it an artefact? The same trials indicated that some of the people who did best on Zelmid had been those who were most suicidal in the early stages.

To produce Zelmid, Astra manipulated the structure of an antihistamine, chlorpheniramine, a potent serotonin reuptake inhibitor, which has since been shown to share many properties of the SSRIs. It treats anxiety and panic attacks. If companies or scientists had simply wanted to see what effects these new compounds might have, they wouldn't have needed to go to the trouble of creating new drugs. But because Zelmid was a new molecule, Astra could take out a patent on it. The patent system offers the possibility of huge returns but brings responsibilities in exchange.

Indalpine and psychiatry under siege

Another manipulation of the antihistamines produced indalpine, first developed by Gerard le Fur in a French company, Fournier Frères, later part of Rhône Poulenc. After clinical trials, indalpine was marketed in France and other European countries as Upstene, arriving just after Zelmid. It was greeted enthusiastically because it seemed to benefit patients who hadn't responded to other drugs.

But indalpine also ran into trouble. Clinical trials suggested it might lower white blood cell counts. This happens transiently with many psychotropic drugs and for the most part is not a serious problem, although in rare cases, if undetected, it can prove fatal. But to general astonishment, indalpine was removed from the market.

French psychiatrists lobbied the company and the government on behalf of the drug. The experience of Pierre Lambert from Lyon was typical. He and his colleagues had investigated more psychotropic drugs than any other group in either Europe or America,[14] and they believed in indalpine. This was symbolized for them in the suicide of one of their patients. Chronically depressed, she had been transformed by indalpine. When the drug was withdrawn from the market, she relapsed. Nothing else appeared to make any difference. She kept going in the hope that the drug might be restored to the market, but when it wasn't, she committed suicide. Her suicide note asked that instead of flowers, a headstone or anything else at her funeral, a collection should be made for medical research. Her family donated the suicide letter and the proceeds of the collection to research.

There was another factor that influenced Rhône Poulenc. A range of what were first termed ecologist or green groups and later pharmacovigilance groups had emerged in Germany in the 1970s, some of which had started in the context of the antipsychiatry protests of the late 1960s. They argued against physical therapies in psychiatry. Campaigning by such groups led to electroconvulsive therapy (ECT) being banned in a number of countries. Psychiatry was under siege. The neutropenia that indalpine caused made it a target for these new pharmacovigilantes.

Emboldened by the demise of indalpine, the new pharmacovigilantes set their sights on another antidepressant, nomifensine, a dopamine reuptake inhibitor, which in a number of cases had triggered hemolytic anemia. They were successful, and nomifensine was also withdrawn. In the face of this onslaught from "fringe groups," European psychiatrists dug in. This was not a matter of protecting the pharmaceutical industry, but of losing useful tools. At the time, there were then no other drugs like indalpine or nomifensine on the market.

The next target for the pharmacovigilantes was mianserin, the best-selling antidepressant in Europe. Like indalpine, mianserin could lower white cell counts. In response to letters pointing out that mianserin could trigger this potentially fatal problem, Roger Pinder, a senior scientist at Organon, its maker, responded that all the antidepressants then available *except* mianserin could be lethal in overdose, so that even if some people did die from white cell problems, overall fewer would die using mianserin than any other antidepressant. The response from the critics was that suicide was illegal.

Organon's defence worked across Europe except in Britain, where the regulator wanted mianserin withdrawn. Organon made it clear that it was prepared to take the matter all the way to the European Court. This situation was unprecedented. In the ordinary course of events, a company faced with regulatory disapproval would simply comply. Eventually Organon won, but the disputes led to a collapse of mianserin sales[15]. The company replaced it with mirtazapine (Remeron), an almost identical molecule.

Organon's safety in overdose argument became a key card played by Lilly in its arguments with the regulators over the safety of Prozac. This argument was new to regulators, who were being asked to contemplate a scenario equivalent to the pope being urged to allow condoms on the basis that they minimize the spread of AIDS. The argument was new to regulators, who were faced with the dilemma that letting a drug with a known hazard remain on the market opened them up to legal actions. This was uncharted territory.

The events surrounding indalpine and mianserin put in place a set of jigsaw pieces that gave glimpses of what was later to be the SSRI story, with the Church of Scientology replacing the German Greens as the bogeymen. Suicide was to become an issue in these debates. The network of "friends" Organon mobilized later played a part in managing the controversy over SSRIs and suicide in Europe. Lilly organized a similar network in the United States.

How Luvox came to Columbine

The first SSRI to survive on the world market was fluvoxamine. This was developed in 1973 from another antihistamine and marketed by Duphar Laboratories as Faverin from 1983 in Europe. But in Germany it was held up because in clinical trials there had been a higher number of suicide attempts on fluvoxamine than on comparator drugs.

Duphar was asked to account for this. The company consulted experts around Europe. When the data the regulators saw were reanalysed focusing specifically on those who were most suicidal to begin with, fluvoxamine seemed to reduce suicidality just as much as the comparator drugs imipramine and amitriptyline. The lesson, the company suggested, was that the apparently higher rate of suicide attempts on fluvoxamine was a chance development—in fact SSRIs might prove even more anti-suicidal than older drugs. The "experts" were learning how to handle the regulators on this issue.

In the 1980s, after licensing, new antidepressants were given to patients hospitalized with depression who had been unresponsive to other therapies—not a promising group on which to try a new drug. Fluvoxamine produced poor responses, along with severe nausea in many patients. Its sales remained flat. But another route to salvation opened up.

By general consent, Geigy's clomipramine is the most potent antidepressant. This tricyclic, made in 1958, with potent effects on both the norepinephrine and serotonin system, was the last of the major tricyclic antidepressants to come to market. Many viewed it as just another me-too drug. The FDA was keen to discourage copycat drugs and did not license it.

George Beaumont, a physician with Geigy, learned of reports that clomipramine might help treat obsessive-compulsive disorder (OCD). He organized a series of OCD studies in the early 1970s, saw a positive response to the drug, and got it licensed for the treatment of both depression and OCD in Britain.

Companies had regarded OCD as even less interesting than depression in the 1950s. But by the late 1980s, under the influence of Judith Rapoport's *The Boy who Couldn't Stop Washing* and the success of clomipramine in Europe, OCD looked worth pursuing[16]. Clomipramine was finally licensed in the United States in 1990 for OCD rather than depression. Fluvoxamine, branded as Luvox, followed, also to treat OCD. It was the low-profile SSRI until the killings at Columbine High School in Colorado in 1999, when it was reported that one of the shooters was on Luvox for OCD.

Where SSRIs make some people agitated and suicidal, one of the lessons of later clinical trials like Study 329 on adolescents showed that they tend to make people with obsessive features agitated and homicidal.

Celexa and Lexapro: Danish fairy tale

In 1971, Lundbeck, a Danish pharmaceutical company, hired Klaus Bøgesø as a medicinal chemist. In the game of drug hunting, Bøgesø had a Midas touch.

The challenge facing him after his recruitment was to produce a selective norepinephrine reuptake inhibitor. Like other companies at the time, Lundbeck had little interest in an SSRI.

Bøgesø quickly produced talopram and tasulopram,[17] which were pressed into clinical trials. Both turned out to increase energy levels, and both were linked to a number of suicide attempts. This appeared to confirm one of the major theories of the time that energy-increasing, or activating, antidepressants might lead to suicide. Lundbeck retreated. Suicide was the greatest hazard of an antidepressant. Kielholz's views suggested that less activating antidepressants would be less likely to trigger suicide. His views also suggested that SSRIs were less likely to be activating. Following a lead from Arvid Carlsson, Bøgesø converted talopram into citalopram, the most selective of the serotonin reuptake inhibitors.

The detour through talopram left Lundbeck behind its competitors. Nevertheless, citalopram made it to the Danish market in 1984, three years before Prozac. Lundbeck undercut the cost of the other SSRIs, and promoted citalopram as the most selective SSRI and least likely to cause side effects. It sold well.

In the United States the story was more extraordinary. In January 1998, *The New Yorker* featured an article by Andrew Solomon titled "Anatomy of Melancholy," about the author's own depression. Within a month Solomon received 2,000 letters from other sufferers. Clearly, he had struck a nerve. His article was anthologized in more than 30 books, and he became a spokesperson in forums such as the American Psychiatric Association.

One of the piece's most striking points was his description of the effects of Zoloft as being like drinking 55 cups of black coffee and the effects of Paxil as being the equivalent of 11 cups of black coffee. Users seemed well aware of this stimulating, agitating effect at a time when both manufacturers and clinicians were denying it.

After failing to negotiate a marketing agreement with Pfizer, which was worried about the risk of birth defects, and then with Warner-Lambert, Lundbeck gave up on the U.S. market—until they met Howard Solomon

(Andrew Solomon's father), chief executive of Forest Laboratories. Forest was a marketing rather than a pharmaceutical company. It launched citalopram under the brand name Celexa in September 1998; by undercutting the price of other SSRIs and marketing aggressively, Celexa captured such a large market share that it became front-page news.

A small number of drugs come in mixes of close to identical left and right-handed molecules—such as Astra's omeprazole (Losec) which can be split into esomeprazole (Nexium) and dexomeprazole. Usually one is active and the other inactive. Citalopram was one of these. Its left hand and active part is escitalopram (s is for sinister which means the left hand). Escitalopram is the bit of citalopram that acts when you take citalopram. The patent system is supposed to ensure we get truly novel compounds, but it has become so weak that companies can now take out patents on isomers like escitalopram just before the patent on the parent citalopram has expired. This is what Lundbeck did and both it and Forest marketed escitalopram as Lexapro equally aggressively and successfully.

When concerns blew up about SSRIs causing suicide in children, there was a Forest study of Celexa, authored by Karen Wagner and others of the 329 group, that seemed to paint it as the only SSRI free of the problem. A later study of Lexapro had a similar message. Forest encouraged this interpretation, and the Teamsters' Union invested in company shares. Forest board members were selling their shares at the same time. It later turned out that Lundbeck had run a trial of citalopram in children where it had thrown up one of the highest suicidal act rates seen in any clinical trial. When this emerged, the Forest share price tumbled and the Teamsters took a legal action, which Forest settled. Forest were later charged and fined by the Department of Justice. In 2014 they disappeared into Actavis—a company few had heard of before.

Prozac: the fifth SSRI

In the 1960s Eli Lilly was, in terms of psychiatric drugs, a small pharmaceutical company. Its best-selling antidepressant was nortriptyline, a norepinephrine reuptake inhibitor. In 1971, taking another antihistamine, diphenhydramine as a starting point, Lilly chemist Bryan Molloy came up with a group of phenoxyphenyl-propylamines. Of the 57 chemicals in the group, the one given the code LY-94939, later called nisoxetine, had the profile Lilly was interested in. It was a norepinephrine reuptake inhibitor, and the company moved it into clinical trials.

Lilly had little interest in serotonin. But in line with standard practice, the other compounds in the series were investigated. David Wong, a biochemist, tested all of Molloy's new series and several came out as serotonin inhibitors. LY-82816 stood out as the compound with the least effect on the norepinephrine system. It was difficult to work with, as it couldn't easily be dissolved, so it was reformulated as a chloride salt, becoming LY-110140. At this point, work on LY-110140 was an academic exercise, just about meriting publication in a journal.

As reports of Zelmid's progress came through, Frank Bymaster and Ray Fuller, pharmacologists with the company, looked at LY-110140's effects on behaviour. They screened it for antidepressant activity. The best-known screening test involved trying to block the sedative effects of a drug called reserpine on animals. Reserpine depleted norepinephrine, serotonin and dopamine. All of the antidepressants then on the market blocked reserpine-induced sedation; LY-110140 did not. Another test was a rat aggression model. If a drug made rats more aggressive, conventional wisdom had it that such drugs might be useful in the treatment of depression. LY-110140 increased aggression in rats.

On September 11, 1975, LY-110140 was named fluoxetine. It had a relatively unusual biochemical effect, and some poorly characterized behavioural effects, but otherwise it was a mystery. Carlsson's work suggested it might be useful for treating nerves or depression, but most companies were adopting a wait-and-see attitude to these claims.

Lilly invited a number of clinical investigators to a consultancy meeting in Britain in the late 1970s. One was Alec Coppen, one of the first advocates of the serotonin hypothesis of depression. They were presented with data on a range of Lilly compounds. Coppen suggested that fluoxetine might be an antidepressant, only to be told that if fluoxetine was ever developed, there was little chance it would be for depression[18].

There were a number of other possibilities. Drugs acting on serotonin were antihypertensive in animal models. This was a much bigger market than the antidepressant market. Had fluoxetine shown any antihypertensive action, there is little doubt that it would have been developed as an antihypertensive. The "behavioural effects" would have been written out of the script as the marketing emphasized the rational engineering of a selective antihypertensive, although around this time some ACE-inhibitor antihypertensives, such as Zestril, were in fact marketed as also being mood-enhancing.

There were other lucrative possibilities. Early screening suggested fluoxetine might produce weight loss. An anti-obesity agent was certain to make more money than an antidepressant. The hint that fluoxetine had weight-reducing properties probably drove some of the early mania, which later helped it hit the road running when it was marketed as Prozac in 1989. As late as 1990, the company still hoped to license fluoxetine in a 60-mg pill under the trade name Loban for eating disorders. The vast amounts of money to be made in this market by drugs active on the serotonergic system made Fen-Phen headline news a few years later.

The early Prozac trials were a problem. The first trialist, Herbert Meltzer, had a longstanding interest in the capacity of antipsychotics to cause side effects like *akathisia* (restlessness) and parkinsonism. When one of his patients on fluoxetine became restless, Meltzer was certain the patient had accidentally been given an antipsychotic, but then other patients developed akathisia and a range of problems previously much more commonly linked to antipsychotics than antidepressants. There was little benefit for depression.

Other senior clinicians found something similar. Most centres had patients who became agitated or akathisic. This led to recommendations from Lilly monitors that it would be necessary to give at least some patients benzodiazepines in clinical trials of fluoxetine. A far-reaching implication of this is that there may be no clinical trial in which fluoxetine on its own has ever been shown to be an "antidepressant."

The company persuaded clinicians to try it out in patients with atypical psychotic disorders as well as patients hospitalized with depressive disorders or melancholia. It turned out to be ineffective in both groups. It made patients with psychotic features worse, and it has never been shown to work for hospital depression. Fluoxetine was at a crisis point.

Irwin Slater, a veteran of drug development within the company, was drafted to take over the clinical trials program. He tried fluoxetine out for pain syndromes, obesity and other conditions, with no great luck. Senior management were pushing to shelve the compound, but Slater and Fuller pointed out that Zelmid was almost through a clinical trials program for depression, with Luvox not far behind. The hierarchy relented. A clinical trial program began chasing milder depressions. Louis Fabre, later investigated by Upjohn for "recruiting patients from a half-way house for alcoholics," was approached. He gave fluoxetine to five patients; all "responded." This turned the tide.

With fluoxetine rescued, the next step was to think about how to brand it. Lilly turned to Interbrand, which later claimed it invented the "discipline of naming" in the late 1970s. The success of the name Prozac changed how drugs were named. Prior to Prozac, drugs had names that sounded scientific and referred in some way to the actual compound—like Luvox and Zelmid. But *Prozac* was designed to convey professionalism (the *Pro-* element) and the ability of the medication to target the right area for treatment (the *-zac* element).

Prozac's brush with extinction may have had one long-lasting consequence. Many clinicians wondered why Lilly didn't bring in low doses of Prozac. With a 5-mg dose, some of the problems that emerged at higher doses might have been minimized. The conventional explanation was that Lilly had a brilliant marketing strategy, which involved selling one pill at one dose—something any fool could give.

But the alarming early history of Prozac, the difficulties in showing it worked, meant the company pushed the dose up to 80 mg a day at one point. In the mid-1980s, when the FDA was finding it difficult to be certain Prozac worked at all, a Lilly study demonstrated that for the new mild depression market they were investigating, 5 mg was as effective as 20 or 40 mg. But this was just too tricky a finding to let see the light of day.

Prozac was treading a path between the Scylla of serious depression—where it didn't work—and the Charybdis of mild depression—where the newer antidepressants all seemed to come unstuck. For a time, no new antidepressants made it to the U.S. market, which may have helped Prozac, given that it was the first antidepressant to hit the U.S. market for quite some time.

The trials that finally led to its being licensed included three placebo-controlled studies. Karl Rickels from Philadelphia conducted one; it was negative. A second was a six-centre study, called protocol 27, where Prozac was compared to imipramine and placebo. The data of one of the investigators, Jay Cohn from Los Angeles, were later removed at the request of the FDA because the extremely favourable results were at odds with the rest of the data. When the remaining studies were combined, Prozac was inferior to imipramine and barely better than placebo on some scales, and no better than placebo on others. Three of the six centres failed to show it better than placebo. In the final study, by Louis Fabre, there were only 11 completers on Prozac, and the study period was effectively only four weeks in duration. It came up with a positive result for Prozac. With the Fabre study and counting protocol 27 as one study, the score was two to one in favour of Prozac. If the component centres of the multicentre study are counted separately, the result was four centres in favour of Prozac and four against—hardly an overwhelming majority.

The plan had been to launch Prozac in the United States in 1986. The FDA finally approved it in late 1987, after three years of scrutiny, during which the agency noted serious flaws in its clinical trials.

In line with a strategy developed in 1983, the early sales pitch stressed that Prozac lacked the nasty side effects of the older tricyclics but that it was as efficacious as these drugs and came in a convenient once-daily dosing. Borrowing from the mianserin story, there was an emphasis on safety in overdose. And finally there was an emphasis on weight loss. Right from the time of its launch in the United States, patients began lining up asking for Prozac by name, an experience new to American psychiatrists.

Over the course of the following few years, every company with SSRIs ran clinical trials comparing their drug with the older antidepressants. The companies only published just over half of the trials, and in some cases ghostwriters transformed a negative study of the SSRI into a positive endorsement. When all of these ghostwritten trials were analyzed together, the SSRIs could not be shown to be any more effective in outpatient depressions than the older agents. As for the tolerability profiles of the SSRIs compared with the older drugs, it would take more than 30 patients assigned to either set of drugs before there would be one fewer dropout in the SSRI group. This was the case even though these trials were almost exclusively designed by SSRI companies, so that in over 30% of trials, the SSRI had been pitched against the tricyclic generally thought to have the most side effects—amitriptyline.

The contrast between the marketing hype and the data was extraordinary. The greatest predictor of the outcome of a trial lay in its sponsorship. Later in the decade it became clear that a large number of trials with less favourable results for the SSRIs were simply not reported, and that the results on quality of life scales used in many of these trials were left almost universally unreported.

The trump card for the SSRIs has been that a greater number of patients are likely to be put on and remain on what is thought to be a "therapeutic dose" of a drug than with other agents. But even here, the puzzle is that no more than 40% of patients take their drugs for more than a few weeks. Something goes wrong with the other 60%. This "something" tempts clinicians to blame patients and tempts the "experts" to blame the family doctor, who supposedly hasn't stressed to the patient the importance of remaining on treatment for six months or more. Nowhere is there any concession to the possibility that SSRIs may not suit up to 60% of those put on them.

By the time Prozac got its licence, the crisis with the benzodiazepines had become severe. The psychiatric and family medicine worlds were receptive to the idea that behind every case of anxiety lay a case of depression. No one was inclined to question the idea that antidepressants were a more scientifically rational treatment for the nervous states presenting in the community than anxiolytics, especially when no one then expected an antidepressant to produce dependence. Add in the fact that compared with older antidepressants these new drugs were safe in overdose, and there seemed to be no good reason not to prescribe them.

The plans had been to launch fluoxetine in Germany in 1984, but it took six more years for 'Fluctin' to reach the market there. Probably very few people outside Lilly, Pfizer, and SmithKline Beecham knew the view of German regulators on fluoxetine as of May 1984: "Considering the benefit and the risk, we think this preparation totally unsuitable for the treatment of depression."[19]

Instead, the extraordinary market success of Prozac led Pfizer and SmithKline to speed up the development of Zoloft and Paxil.

Zoloft: the least effective SSRI?

Zoloft began life in 1977. Playing around with some of the original antipsychotics, Pfizer chemists produced a series of norepinephrine reuptake inhibitors, of which tametraline looked the most promising. When side effects halted its development in 1979, Willard Welch transformed it into a series of serotonin reuptake inhibitors, one of which was sertraline.

While the SSRIs were in development, the FDA began to insist that companies would need two placebo-controlled trials if they were going to claim their drug worked. There was an uproar. Many clinical trial programs did not include placebo trials. Worse yet, several new compounds could not be shown to work when compared against placebo. Mianserin, the best-selling antidepressant in Europe, failed in U.S. placebo-controlled trials, perhaps because these trials were conducted in a too mildly depressed group, where it is difficult to demonstrate that *any* antidepressant is superior to placebo.

The ambiguities are most clearly seen in the licence application for Zoloft, where only one of five studies indicated superiority over placebo. A further study claimed superiority for Zoloft when some patients who had their treatment discontinued "relapsed," but in this case what was termed relapse was likely withdrawal from Zoloft. Zoloft did less well than amitriptyline and failed in two hospital depression studies. As Paul Leber, the senior FDA official, ended up putting it:

> *How do we interpret two positive results in the context of several more studies that fail to demonstrate that effect? I am not sure I have an answer to that, but I am not sure that the law requires me to have an answer to that—fortunately or unfortunately. That would mean, in a sense, that the sponsor could just do studies until the cows come home until he gets two of them that are statistically significant by chance alone, walks them out and says he has met the criteria.*[20]

For those who believe that approval of a drug by the FDA means that it is in some sense good for you if taken properly, the situation is even more problematic. "Two positive studies" doesn't mean the drug works for depression in two studies. It means there are two studies in which the drug can be shown to have an effect on depression—can be shown to do *something*. Whether it is a good idea to take any of these drugs is not addressed. These trials do not offer evidence that the drug "works" in the sense that most people mean by the word *works*—that is, evidence of lives saved or people able to return to work.

Companies marketing their products do not have to reveal anything about the weak evidence on which registration was based. The new compound can be sold with all the glossy slogans of rational engineering, hints of added benefits for weight loss or whatever, and celebrity endorsements. Since the end of the 1980s, companies did not have to worry that independent investigators might question just how good their compound really was, as there were vanishingly few independent investigators left in the medical sphere.

If all that is needed is some rating scale changes in short trials for mild to moderate depression, it would be possible to show that alcohol, stimulants and benzodiazepines are "antidepressants." Such trials have been done but the fact no company has applied for a license owes everything to a business calculation: no company stands to make money from drugs that are off-patent.

We are accustomed to the notion that our regulators are looking after us, that they are in some sense a consumer watchdog. But the role of a regulator is to adjudicate whether, for example, a yellow substance in front of her meets minimal criteria to be considered butter; to ensure that it is not, say, lard injected with colour. Regulators are not called upon to determine whether this butter is good butter or not, or whether eating butter is good for your health. Consumer watchdogs must do that. Within medicine, the physician is supposed to be the consumer's watchdog. Given that doctors don't generally consume the product, this makes for an ambiguous and commercially unique situation.

The legal situation is even more complex. If the regulators' mandate is to let drugs onto the market that are *proven to have an effect*, what the FDA has been doing is defensible. If the task, as per the wording of the statutes in most countries, is to license drugs that are *effective*, then it is much less sure that the SSRIs have been proven to be effective.

Despite having close to no evidence of benefit, sertraline launched as Zoloft in 1991. Pfizer emphasized technical differences between it and the other SSRIs—claiming that it had a better half-life, cleaner metabolism and a lower liability to interact with other compounds in the body, making it safer than other SSRIs. This strategy produced the appearances of science—lots of data—but few of these data were clinically relevant. The approach was geared to making Zoloft appear "clean" compared with Prozac and Paxil. The other companies responded, leading to a "War between the Sisters," which helped make Zoloft a blockbuster.

Paxil and the spectre of dependence

Paroxetine was developed in 1978 by Jorgen Buus-Lassen, who worked for a small Danish company called Ferrosan. In 1975, he had produced an earlier SSRI, femoxetine, which appeared more effective than paroxetine but had the disadvantage of not being a simple once-a-day pill.

In 1980 Ferrosan sold paroxetine to Beecham Pharmaceuticals, which later merged with SmithKline & French to become SmithKline Beecham (SB). SB merged again with Glaxo in 2000 to become GlaxoSmithKline (GSK), at that point the world's largest pharmaceutical corporation. Ferrosan was acquired by Novo-Nordisk, which had little interest in psychiatry, and so femoxetine died from neglect.

Paroxetine nearly died of neglect as well. Beecham was considering shelving it because it appeared less effective than older antidepressants. A Danish Universities Antidepressant Group study confirmed this.[21] This was at a time when the non-hospital depression market still appeared relatively small, so it was not obvious how a less effective antidepressant could be expected to make much money. As a result of company ambivalence, the clinical development of paroxetine lagged behind that of Zelmid, and later Prozac.

Paroxetine was licensed as Paxil in the United States in 1992 and as Seroxat in the United Kingdom in 1991. SmithKline marketing coined the acronym SSRI. Compared to the other serotonin reuptake inhibitors, paroxetine was supposedly the selective serotonin reuptake inhibitor. This was far from the truth, but the name worked all too well and was adopted for the entire group of compounds. Thus Paxil made Prozac and Zoloft into SSRIs.

The idea of an SSRI conveys the impression of a clean and specific drug, freer from side effects than the non-selective tricyclic antidepressants. However, selectivity for pharmacologists meant that an SSRI could act on every brain system except the norepinephrine system. It was selective away from norepinephrine. The SSRIs could be dirtier drugs than the tricyclics and still be selective. Clinicians were misled by this marketing, which suggested "selective" meant these drugs went directly to one targeted area, like the mythical Magic Bullet.

Chasing Prozac, SmithKline targeted anxiety—panic disorder, anxious depressions, generalized anxiety disorder, post-traumatic stress disorder (PTSD) and later social phobia. This targeting led to huge sales, making Paxil the closest rival to Prozac. In 2001, when Prozac went off-patent, Paxil surpassed it in sales.

When GSK obtained a licence to market Paxil for social phobia, its stock rose—an anti-shyness pill was potentially a huge market. While widely recognized in Japan and Korea, social phobia had until 1990 been almost unknown in the Western world. It was first described in the 1960s in London by Isaac Marks. There is an obvious overlap between social phobia and shyness and a risk therefore that legitimate efforts to market a treatment for a disabling medical condition will at the same time capture a significant number of people who are simply shy—and who may be at more risk from the treatment than from their shyness. The marketing by SmithKline, assisted by the opening up of direct-to-consumer advertising, appeared geared to anyone with shyness. The term social phobia suggests that the appropriate treatment is a behaviour therapy. This apparently did not suit SmithKline; in response in the 1990s, organized psychiatry rolled over and replaced "social phobia" with "social anxiety disorder."

While hugely successful in terms of sales, the targeting of Paxil for anxiety disorders contained a snag. Soon after its launch, primary care physicians and others began to describe dependence on SSRIs through adverse event reporting systems.[22] There was a much greater volume of reports for Paxil than for other SSRIs. The first suggestion was that these withdrawal effects stemmed from Paxil's short half-life—something SmithKline was marketing as a safety feature. In response to claims of dependence, it was then suggested that as Paxil was used more than other SSRIs to treat anxiety, perhaps any problems had to do with the personalities of these patients, who were after all more likely than others to develop phobias—why not a withdrawal phobia?

Amid reports of withdrawal symptoms in the mid-1990s, Lilly convened a panel of "opinion leaders" to discuss what were termed "antidepressant discontinuation syndromes" rather than dependence problems. This was quite cynical in that Prozac had a very long half-life, so that while it might also cause these problems, because of its half-life the problem was less likely to show.[23] Sensing a market opportunity vis-à-vis Paxil and Zoloft, Lilly began to run advertisements about discontinuation syndromes.

In so doing, Lilly brought the spectre of dependence back to the table. A key reason to develop SSRIs as antidepressants lay in the fact that clinicians suspected all tranquilizers would in due course produce dependence, just as the benzodiazepines had done. In the early 1990s, doctors did not associate the antidepressants with dependence. But when the Royal College of Psychiatrists launched its *Defeat Depression* campaign in 1992 and engaged professional polling organizations, it found that the public thought antidepressants were likely to be addictive. The College went out of its way to counter this perception, and most clinicians felt comfortable saying these drugs did not produce addiction or dependence. The backs of Prozac packets actually contain an explicit statement: "Don't worry about taking Prozac over a long period of time—Prozac is not addictive."

If by *addictive* we mean that the drug will transform those taking it into junkies, likely to mortgage their livelihoods and futures for an ongoing supply of drugs, then the SSRIs do not appear to be addictive. They do not lead to a life of crime or dissolution. But this does not mean SSRIs don't produce dependence. Many people experience grave difficulties in discontinuing treatment from Paxil or Zoloft. In lay terms, you can just as easily become hooked on SSRIs as on benzodiazepines or opiates, and SSRIs can be more difficult to get off than anything else. For most of us this is the meaning of addiction.

With the SSRIs, a problem called poop-out was noted early on. Poop-out refers to the drugs losing their effect; sometimes they can be got to work again by increasing the dose. This phenomenon first came to light in internet chat rooms rather than through physicians being informed by drug companies of a problem. Because the companies in fact denied the problem, doctors could not advise on the best means of managing it; clinicians were left to their own devices. This is hardly the kind of partnership that is supposed to characterize prescription-only arrangements.

Whereas suicide while taking an SSRI is something most people find hard to envisage happening to them, we can all envisage getting hooked on a drug and remaining alive to complain about it. But in 2001, when Prozac went off-patent, Paxil's fortunes still looked good. It was the number one selling antidepressant in the world; in addition, the Keller et al. Study 329 paper had just appeared, opening up a huge new market.

Managed non-selectivity

Venlafaxine (Efexor) tagged along several years behind Prozac, Paxil and Zoloft. Even though at doses of up to 150 mg per day—four times the initial starting dose—this drug was primarily a selective serotonin reuptake inhibitor, the branding strategy adopted was to call it a serotonergic and noradrenergic reuptake inhibitor—an SNRI. This is just marketing copy—it has no scientific meaning. Efexor did modestly well in terms of sales, in part because it caused significant dependence and once on it patients risked becoming customers for life. As a serotonin reuptake inhibitor, it caused all the agitation these drugs caused, especially in children.

Like Celexa, venlafaxine came in isomer form, and when it went off-patent the company brought desvenlafaxine (Pristiq), the active component of venlafaxine with an identical profile of actions, onto the market. There should be no rationale for clinicians to prescribe the more expensive Pristiq rather than the off-patent venlafaxine but doctors have no more discrimination when it comes to branded products than teenage boys do.

Like Celexa and Efexor, Prozac too came as isomers—dexfluoxetine and s-fluoxetine. In this case both isomers were active. The initial plan when Prozac went off-patent was to replace it with s-fluoxetine, but these plans were shelved, and Lilly turned to dexfluoxetine, which had been isolated and patented by a company called Sepracor, on the basis that it was less likely to cause risky agitation than the parent Prozac.

Dexfluoxetine was branded as Zalutria and was due to launch. The marketing plans were developed. The trial data were with the FDA. Then Lilly suddenly withdrew it. The explanation given was that it caused QT-interval problems—cardiac effects—which might lead to sudden death. But if Zalutria causes this, which it almost certainly does, then Prozac must—and does—do the same thing.

Lilly were left scraping the end of the barrel. They had developed a norepinephrine reuptake inhibitor, atomoxetine, but decided that this would not qualify as an antidepressant. On the basis of its effects on John Heiligenstein, a company employee, it was brought on the market instead as Strattera, the first non-dependence producing treatment for attention deficit hyperactivity disorder (ADHD). It was later marketed heavily for adult ADHD—or rather adult ADHD was marketed to bring patients to it.

Lilly had another option—a drug called duloxetine. The "dual" in duloxetine refers to the fact that it inhibits the reuptake of both serotonin and norepinephrine. It is a more straightforward SNRI than Efexor was. But in line with other companies who developed drugs like this in the mid-1990s, Lilly had junked plans to develop duloxetine as an antidepressant. The company line at the time was that it caused side effects. Among the main side effects was urinary retention. This action led to its development as a bladder stabilizer, and it came on the market in Europe for this purpose. Efforts to get it marketed for bladder stabilization in the United States failed when the FDA decided that it was causing too many suicidal events in healthy women.

But ultimately it came onto the U.S. market as an antidepressant under the trade name Cymbalta. In any rational market, Cymbalta should never have gotten anywhere, but all too predictably it became a $3 billion blockbuster, earning more than Prozac did in its heyday. Key to the marketing success was its badging as also effective for pain. This was just when the pain-killer Vioxx ran into trouble. Physicians were looking around for a safe painkiller and seized on Cymbalta, unaware that this was an off the peg marketing campaign originally developed for Zalutria. There was no substantive reason to think Cymbalta was any better for pain relief than Prozac.

CHAPTER 5

The Suicide Controversies

Long before Shelley Jofre helped create a controversy about antidepressants and suicide, the problem had bucked like a bull in a rodeo. But in 2002, as she flew to Philadelphia, the companies and FDA looked comfortably seated in the saddle.

The psychopharmacological era began in 1952 when reserpine and chlorpromazine were both reported to have benefits in psychosis. Initially there was no such thing as an antipsychotic or antidepressant, partly because both reserpine and chlorpromazine looked as if they might be useful for all nervous problems. Chlorpromazine sold in Europe under the trade name Largactil, which point to a large action—it worked for everything from itch and nausea to anxiety and psychosis. Reserpine, sold as Serpasil, was the first to be called a tranquilizer. When Librium and Valium hijacked this new term, reserpine and chlorpromazine became the major tranquilizers in contrast to the benzodiazepine minor tranquilizers.

There was every reason to believe that reserpine in lower doses might help anxiety or depression. This led Michael Shepherd to undertake the first modern clinical trial in psychiatry in which he compared reserpine to placebo in a group of anxious depressives[24]. In Shepherd's study, published in 1955, reserpine in fact showed better results as an antidepressant than later results for SSRIs in similar patient groups. But Ciba, the makers of Serpasil, weren't interested in an antidepressant.

In 1955, another reserpine paper created neuroscience. In this, Steve Brodie at the NIH demonstrated reserpine both sedated rabbits and at the same time lowered their brain serotonin levels[25]. This was the first demonstration of a link between brain chemistry and behaviour. Pharmacologists from around the world flocked to work with Brodie, including the creator of the SSRIs, Arvid Carlsson, who among other things showed that reserpine also lowered both norepinephrine and dopamine.

The first controversy

In the early 1950s, reserpine was primarily used as an antihypertensive. A number of physicians noted that hypertensive patients taking it reported feeling "better than well." In 1954, Robert Wilkins claimed physicians were suggesting it was time to give up psychotherapy, as reserpine was good psychotherapy in pill form.[26]

But starting in 1955, a series of reports emerged of hypertensive patients becoming "depressed" on reserpine and committing suicide. Both it and chlorpromazine could make some patients feel flat and demotivated, but in contrast to proper depression this problem cleared up once the drug was stopped or if the patient was given a stimulant.

But reserpine also did more of something else. In the first paper to describe hypertensive patients becoming suicidal, Richard Achor from the Mayo Clinic reported that it caused some patients "increased tenseness, restlessness, insomnia, and a feeling of being very uncomfortable." Robert Faucett gave further details: "The first few doses frequently made them anxious and apprehensive... They reported increased feelings of strangeness, verbalized by statements such as 'I don't feel like myself'... or 'I'm afraid of some of the unusual impulses that I have.'" Gerald Sarwer-Foner described a subject who on the first day of treatment reacted with marked anxiety and weeping and on the second day "felt so terrible with such marked panic at night that the medication was cancelled."

This is not depression. This is akathisia. Akathisia literally means an inability to sit still. It was first noted following brain injuries and then in the encephalitis lethargica epidemic of 1918. Encephalitis lethargica produced instant Parkinson's disease in some, rendering them mute and stuporous, but it made others restless and agitated. The antipsychotics also cause parkinsonism and akathisia—none more so than reserpine.

Akathisia is one of the least understood pieces of medical jargon. The best translation into English is mental turmoil or agitation. It produces an inner restlessness, with outer restlessness in some cases too, which has led some people to think it's a motor disorder. It's not. When the problem began to show up in company trials of the SSRIs in the 1980s, it was coded as agitation—and as restlessness, hyperactivity, anxiety, and depression. The multiple ways it can be coded hid it in plain sight.

It is often said a psychiatric drug can never be shown to cause suicide because patients are already at risk of suicide from their original nervous condition. But none of the reports of suicide on reserpine were in people with a nervous problem—they were all hypertensive. As other antihypertensives and antipsychotics emerged, reserpine was shelved. This was partly because it was available off-patent and so no company had an incentive to defend it, in contrast to other antipsychotics and later SSRIs when they caused the same problems.

Unaware that reserpine had been shown to be an antidepressant, Joe Schildkraut used its capacity to lower norepinephrine levels as a key element in his theory of depression. Everyone agreed, he claimed, that reserpine could trigger depression and suicides. It did this, he argued, by lowering norepinephrine levels, and therefore depression involved low norepinephrine.

Then in 1958, imipramine launched as the first tricyclic antidepressant. It was much more potent clinically than later SSRIs. It brought about recoveries in melancholic patients who would otherwise have been expected to respond only to electroconvulsive therapy. At this point, while ECT was protective against suicide by getting people at high risk of suicide well, it was also linked to suicides in melancholic patients as they came out of their depressive stupor. This was called the rollback phenomenon. The idea was that people were activated and were able to commit suicide before their thinking caught up.

As interest in imipramine grew, a meeting of psychiatrists from all over

Europe was convened in Cambridge, England, in 1959 to share their experiences. Amid general praise for this new treatment, there were several clinicians who noted that it could induce suicidality and aggression in some patients. This problem cleared when the drug was stopped, clearly indicating that it was caused by the drug[27]. The psychiatrists describing what happened on imipramine made it clear that this was not the rollback phenomenon: imipramine could directly agitate some patients.

Depression at this point was a rare disorder and its treatment was mainly hospital-based, so in contrast to what happened with day-care hypertensive patients treated with reserpine, these specialists were comfortable treating a condition that could lead to suicide with a drug that could lead to suicide—good monitoring in hospital would handle most problems.

Meanwhile chlorpromazine and other antipsychotics began to be given to ever increasing numbers of patients with schizophrenia. The suicide rate for schizophrenia climbed twenty-fold between 1955 and 1980. By 1990, this illness which had not been linked to suicide, in contrast to melancholia which was linked, was widely viewed as posing as great a risk of suicide as melancholia. Antipsychotics cause suicide by triggering akathisia[28].

Company suicide or patient suicide?

As of 1985, European regulatory authorities had been faced with several drugs—Zelmid, Luvox and Prozac—showing significant negative side effects, including hallucinations, akathisia, psychosis, agitation and suicidality.

Prozac was approved by FDA on December 29, 1987. It launched in 1988. In December 1989, *New York* magazine published a cover article titled "Bye Bye Blues" about Prozac, calling it a "wonder drug" for depression, weight problems, anxiety, PMS and nicotine withdrawal. The article was unremittingly positive: "Given the number of people taking Prozac and the absence of problems so far, most physicians are impressed."

Two months later in the *American Journal of Psychiatry,* Martin Teicher, Carole Glod and Jonathan Cole, in an article titled "Emergence of Intense Suicidal Preoccupation During Fluoxetine Treatment," reported that "six depressed patients free of recent serious suicidal ideation developed intense, violent suicidal preoccupation after 2–7 weeks of fluoxetine treatment.[29] This state persisted for as little as 3 days to as long as 3 months after discontinuation of fluoxetine. None of these patients had ever experienced a similar state during treatment with any other psychotropic drug."

Across the United States, Prozac Survivors Support Groups formed to help people harmed by Prozac. In May 1991, the FDA noted that since it was marketed in 1988, Prozac (fluoxetine) had had the highest number of adverse event reports submitted to its Adverse Drug Reaction Database. The experts put the reporting down to media bias. The FDA discussed with Lilly a clinical trial specially designed to see whether Prozac was in fact linked to suicidality. The lawyers, including a Santa Monica firm, Baum Hedlund, began to investigate.

In 1991, Mark Riddle and colleagues at Yale University also reported on six children being treated with Prozac for OCD who had become suicidal:

- After five weeks of treatment one of the subjects experienced "very real" violent nightmares about killing his classmates, from which he found it difficult to awaken. He had to be hospitalized. His Prozac was stopped and over several weeks he settled. When restarted on Prozac, his suicidal ideation returned.
- One 14-year-old girl on Prozac began to ruminate about suicide and to bring a knife to school. When her Prozac was increased, her suicidality got worse.
- Another 14-year-old girl became suicidal and agitated on Prozac. She was switched to imipramine, which didn't help. When she was changed back to Prozac, she became violently suicidal. She had to be transferred to a longer-term unit, where she remained significantly suicidal until all antidepressants were stopped.
- Yet another 14-year-old girl, who had initially responded well to Prozac at 20 mg per day, made a first suicide attempt after several months of treatment. Her Prozac was increased to 40 mg per day, and

> over the next two weeks she began pulling out her hair, biting her nails, hitting her legs and requiring restraint:[30].

This paper described the development of intense suicidal ideation on Prozac, which recurred on re-exposure to the drug. Increasing dosages led to the emergence of the problem, where lower doses did not. The pattern was one of a Prozac-induced disturbance emerging during the first few weeks of treatment or shortly after an increase in dose.

Internal Lilly documents from the period show a company frantically scrambling to manage the crisis. The strategy was to blame the disease, not the drug, and to suggest that any legal actions were part of a conspiracy against organized psychiatry by the Church of Scientology. It was critically important to make this work because from inside Lilly it looked like the company was going down the tubes if Prozac went down.

Managing the crisis

In August 1990, Pfizer submitted a portfolio of trials on sertraline to the FDA as part of a new drug application to get Zoloft approved. In 1991, Zoloft was approved by the FDA despite wafer-thin evidence of efficacy in the trials undertaken. The trial data also showed an up to threefold greater risk of suicidal acts on Zoloft compared to a placebo. These data were not brought to the Psychopharmacologic Drugs Advisory Committee (PDAC) hearing devoted to Zoloft's licensing.[31]

On June 19, 1991, SmithKline submitted a new drug application for paroxetine (Paxil). It was reviewed by Martin Brecher, who stated, "Together the safety and efficacy data allow for the conclusion that paroxetine is safe and efficacious and approvable for marketing." At a later PDAC hearing, Tom Laughren of FDA stated, "The safety and efficacy findings for paroxetine were presented to the PDAC on this date (10-5-92), and they unanimously agreed that Paroxetine has been demonstrated to be safe and effective." The data reported in the review show a rate of suicidal acts that is 2.5 times higher in the Paxil group than in the placebo group, but the presentation hid this fact.

The Zoloft and Paxil data were kept hermetically sealed from each other and from the Prozac data, and from the reviewers of Paxil or Zoloft and from the special PDAC set up by the FDA to review the topic of antidepressants and suicide.

On September 20, 1991, the FDA convened a PDAC hearing on the resolution that "there is credible evidence to support a conclusion that SSRI antidepressant drugs cause the emergence and/or intensification of suicidality and/or other violent behaviors." Prozac was the only SSRI considered. The public had not been exposed to Paxil or Zoloft at this point and was unaware of the possibility of an SSRI issue rather than just a Prozac issue. There was no Luvox or Zelmid in the United States. Despite a day of testimony from many people who had experienced Prozac-induced tragedies of violence and suicide, testimony the regulators claimed to find compelling, the committee voted against the resolution. It also voted against warnings for SSRIs on the basis that warnings might deter people from seeking treatment.

Lilly's data were presented to the committee by Charles Nemeroff, whom many there would have seen as friendly but lightweight. The data were also published by the *British Medical Journal (BMJ)* in an article by Charles Beasley, on the same day as the meeting, with the publication circulated at the meeting.[32] Publication in the *BMJ* probably convinced many that the claims in the article that there was no problem must be right. No one would have known that the *BMJ* reviewer pointed to a clear excess of suicidal acts on Prozac compared to the placebo and saw the drug as problematic. But the editor of the *BMJ*, Richard Smith, a fan of the emerging evidence-based medicine, opted to publish. Closer scrutiny of this article shows that key data on Prozac were hidden; the Beasley paper in fact shows Prozac causes suicidal events.

Around the time of the PDAC meeting in September 1991 Prozac and suicide was big news, and there was concerted pressure to sort out the problem. The message that was developed was that anecdotes suggested a problem, but the clinical trial evidence didn't back this up. Are you going to believe the anecdotes or the science? This message laid the panic to rest.

There was a lot of sharp practice involved. There was statistical juggling of trial data by all the companies, and a recoding of suicide events, which went undetected by journalists and others watching what was happening. The juggling was noted by the FDA as being in breach of regulations, but FDA did nothing about it. The FDA exhibited extraordinary compartmentalization in keeping the Zoloft and Paxil data out of the frame, but a decade later it exhibited even greater compartmentalization when it licensed Cymbalta for depression without warnings while refusing to license the same drug for urinary retention on the basis that it provoked suicidality.

Perhaps the most chilling compartmentalization involved the use of Zoloft for children. Pfizer jumped ahead of other companies in exploring the possibility of getting Zoloft on the market for children. They hit on the idea of pushing forward with trials in pediatric OCD. It's easier to demonstrate a benefit for an SSRI in OCD than depression. Pfizer submitted the data to the FDA in December 1995. But James Knudson of FDA wrote to the company in March 1996, asking it to explain an apparently very clear increase in the risk of suicide. Ultimately, however, the company didn't have to. Another FDA official, Tom Laughren, weighed in with a letter saying he didn't think the signal meant anything.

Four years later, in a legal case involving the suicide of 13-year-old Matt Miller, Andy Vickery, the lawyer for the Miller family, deposed Wilma Harrison of Pfizer. Having established that Harrison and Pfizer had every confidence in their investigators, Vickery turned to its OCD studies, picking out the case of an eight-year-old boy who was part of a study that involved pushing the dose of Zoloft up to 200 mg. Vickery asked:[33]

> QUESTION: *An eight-year-old boy who was on Zoloft for 36 days and here's what it says about him: "Patient was hospitalized for a suicide gesture, and dropped from the study. The patient mutilated himself by cutting his feet with a razor blade and tying a tie around his neck. There was no previous history of self-mutilation or suicidality, although family history was significant for affective disorder (mother, maternal uncle) and*

suicide (maternal uncle). The event was attributed to study drug by the investigator.

What does that last sentence mean to you?

ANSWER: *I would like to see the report.*

QUESTION: *The question is: What does the last sentence mean to you?*

ANSWER: *I can only answer that in context. This is a patient who was in a study because the patient had major depression, and the patient has a strong family history of both depression and suicide, so this is a patient that's at very high risk for developing suicidal ideation or behavior.*

The patient was in the study, and the time in the study was probably not sufficient to completely treat the symptoms of depression, so the fact that this patient made a suicide gesture while being treated says that the patient probably was still depressed and feeling suicidal at the time that the patient committed the suicidal gesture.

Now, in order to attribute it to the study drug, I don't see how anybody could attribute it to the study drug. While it's a possibility that you could say that it could be attributed to the study drug, the illness itself is associated with suicidal ideation and behavior, so it is more likely that this patient had made a suicidal gesture because of the underlying depression that was not yet treated.

QUESTION: *That's not what your investigator concluded, is it?*

ANSWER: *I'm a psychiatrist, and I have to assess each case on the basis of facts given to me.*

QUESTION: *You're not going to tell me that you know the eight-year-old boy, are you?*

ANSWER: *I know about treating patients with depression, and, in my clinical judgment, I would not have attributed this to the drug under study. I would have attributed it to the illness under study.*

QUESTION: *Do you know anything about this eight-year-old boy?*

ANSWER: *It is not necessary for me to know about this specific eight-year-old boy. You have given me the history of a family history of affective disorder, a child only eight years old who has a serious enough depression to warrant treatment, and a family history of suicidality. That's very strong risk factors for suicidal behavior.*

QUESTION: *What did Pfizer's clinical investigator conclude with respect to the cause of this boy's suicidal attempt?*

ANSWER: *The investigator attributed it to the study drug.*

The world knew nothing about any of this. The FDA approved Zoloft on December 30, 1991, and Paxil in December 1992 for major depressive disorder (MDD) in adults. The issue of suicide for patients on antidepressants went away until it briefly flickered back onto the radar in 1994 with a legal case against Lilly and Prozac involving mass homicide.

Nor did the world realize that from 1988 onward, the combined clinical trial literature on SSRIs showed a doubling of the rate of suicidal acts on SSRIs compared to placebo; it has stayed that way every year for the last 30 years.[34]

The *Fentress* and *Forsyth* trials

In 1989, Joseph Wesbecker, after two weeks on Prozac prescribed by his physician despite a prior bad reaction to the drug, went to the print shop where he worked armed with an AK-47 and shot and wounded 12 people, killed eight and then turned the gun on himself. Five years later, on September 28, 1994, a trial relating to this incident, *Joyce Fentress et al. vs Eli Lilly,* commenced in Louisville, Kentucky.[35]

Wesbecker offered Lilly a perfect opportunity to play the "it's the disease, not the drug" card. Here was a man with an extensive psychiatric history, including a suicide attempt five years earlier—an accident waiting to happen. He came from a family with three generations of nervous troubles. In building their argument, Lilly's attorneys deposed 400 people, making Wesbecker, as one witness put it, "one of the most studied serial killers in history."

Nancy Lord, an expert for the plaintiffs, brought out many of the issues that later feature in Study 329:

> *When I looked at the Lilly data, I didn't find it was adequate to study this drug. The data was flawed for a number of reasons. First of all, the protocols were not well designed... Not only did they permit the use of concomitant medications, but they permitted the use of psychotropic concomitant medications... If someone came on to a trial and got, say, insomnia, they couldn't sleep, or they became jumpy and agitated, instead of having them withdraw and counting that person as someone who couldn't handle the drug, they simply gave them Dalmane to go to sleep, which had a lingering anxiolytic effect during the next day[36]...*
>
> *It looked like they did everything possible to kind of tone down the problems with the drug rather than give them a rigorous, systematic and comprehensive evaluation to define what the problems were and then put it in the package insert so that doctors could be warned not to use the drug in certain types of patients, or to use it more carefully[37]...*
>
> *In my opinion, this drug has not been approved. It's been approved with sedatives, but taking fluoxetine all by itself has never been studied.[38]*

Some patients in the trials were recorded as having severe agitation but in the summaries of side effects this became nervousness, or was not recorded as a drug side effect "as the investigators were instructed not to record as adverse experience symptoms of depression."[39] Patients who dropped out because of "patient decision" were not followed up to establish whether it was demands on their time or agitation on the drug that had led to their dropping out. A number of patients who had clearly gotten worse on Prozac were deemed to be "treatment non-responders rather than sufferers from side effects of the drug. This pattern had begun from the very first trials, with patients who became severely agitated, suicidal and psychotic being classified as treatment non-responders. Yet when Lilly was approached by investigators wondering how to handle emerging side effects, one of the options suggested was to reduce the dose of Prozac—an option that concedes a causal link between the symptoms and Prozac.

Today the statistical analysis of clinical trials would be done according to a plan put in place before the trials began, but this didn't happen with Prozac. Investigators in many cases were allowed to break the blind and put patients who had done well on Prozac onto maintenance treatment with it, or switch those who had done poorly on imipramine, for instance, to maintenance treatment with Prozac. Maintaining a group of patients on Prozac in this way makes it possible then to claim that when the company controlled for length of exposure on the drug, there wasn't a hazard. In this case patients with the early-onset side effects that Teicher, Glod and Cole had linked to Prozac became diluted by the addition of a selected group of favorable responders to Prozac.

When patients did poorly on Prozac, after a certain number of weeks off Prozac all possible drug-induced difficulties were coded under whatever other drug the patient might then be taking. On the surface this might seem reasonable. After all, if a patient has been off Prozac for some months and is having difficulties, should these be put down to previous Prozac use?

But it is far from reasonable. The rate of suicidal acts on placebo or other antidepressants in Prozac trials is less than 5 per 1,000 patients, while the rate on Prozac is 10 per 1,000. Now suppose the records of 1,000 patients are tracked after they go off Prozac and only those who have problems are recorded. If five of these have a suicidal act and are added to the non-Prozac group, this instantly pushes up the non-Prozac rate to approaching 10 in 1,005—identical to the Prozac rate.[40] The sicker the patients are or the more likely they are to have drug-induced side effects, the more likely they are to stay in contact with the services and be recorded this way.

It was difficult to know what impact Nancy Lord's highly technical testimony might have had on a jury. It was easy for Lilly to appeal to the fact that the FDA had approved this drug, with the implication that FDA officials having considered all these points were nevertheless content to approve Prozac. Can anyone expect a jury of laypeople to find the FDA guilty?

In January 1995, the jury in *Fentress* returned a verdict of 9 to 3 for Lilly. Chief Executive Randall Tobias said, "The members of the jury, after hearing the scientific and medical facts... came to the only logical conclusion—that Prozac had nothing to do with Joseph Wesbecker's actions."[41] Lilly's public relations officer, Ed West, indicated how the verdict would be seen: "If it becomes apparent it's very difficult to win big money in Prozac suits, this probably sends out a message." West added a statement from Tobias that "the verdict demonstrates the futility of blaming medications for harmful and criminal acts."[42]

(In May of 1994, a few months before the trial, Marilyn Tobias, the wife of Randall had died from suicide, shortly after being put on Prozac. Ten years later Tobias was appointed to the role of Global AIDS coordinator for the US government where he ran a program that would disburse money to organizations opposed to prostitution and sex trafficking, saying. "I don't think it's too difficult for people to be opposed to prostitution and sex trafficking, which are in fact two contributing causes to the spread of HIV/AIDS". He resigned on April 27th 2007, Wesbecker's birthday, after being caught using escort services.

Kathryn Taurel, the wife of the CEO succeeding Tobias, Sydney Taurel may also have died by suicide).

Meanwhile, the *Fentress* judge, John Potter, suspected the case had been settled behind the scenes, and filed a motion to change his own post-trial order from "dismissed after verdict" to "dismissed as settled." This made Potter a defendant, but also stopped Lilly's public declarations of exoneration.

On May 23, 1996, the Supreme Court of Kentucky in the case of *Hon. John W. Potter vs Eli Lilly* decided unanimously in Potter's favor, citing the lawyers' serious lack of candor, evidence of bad faith, abuse of process and fraud. Lilly, it appears, had agreed to settle the trial, in exchange for plaintiff lawyers refraining from introducing evidence of other problems Lilly tried to hide.

The attorney for the plaintiffs, Paul Smith, was shunned by the plaintiff's bar afterwards and effectively never worked again. There were several hundred Prozac cases in the pipeline at the time of the *Fentress* trial. But as West predicted, with the verdict for Lilly, they melted away.

While most cases melted away, the Forsyth case didn't. The children of William Forsyth didn't need the money. Their father who had no mental health history was having marital difficulties and wanted to move back from Hawaii to California. His physician gave him Prozac. He became agitated and had to be admitted to hospital. The hospital staff had no idea of the risk when, in a state of restlessness, he then wanted to go home. A day after being discharged, and ten days after going on Prozac, he killed his wife and then himself in what must have been a frenzy. The police attending the scene said they had never seen so much blood. The trial took place in March 1999 in Hawaii. The verdict was again in favor of Lilly and Prozac, but as with the *Fentress* verdict, irregularities came to light after the trial, leading to an appeal and a settlement.

Part of the evidence presented in the appeal, *Forsyth II*, included evidence that Lilly had bought the rights to dex-fluoxetine, patented on the basis that it was less likely to cause suicide than the parent compound.

By 1999, however, the *Fentress* and *Forsyth* settlements were nonevents as far as the public was concerned. The controversies about SSRIs and suicide had been buried even though the *Forsyth* trial released a raft of documents into the public domain showing the concerns of regulators, company efforts to hide data and efforts to frame the problem as an attack by the Church of Scientology on psychiatry. Richard Smith, still the editor of *BMJ* at this point, was given the documents and offered an article on the failure to warn but turned it down flat, saying that no matter what information he was to receive on Prozac, *BMJ* would never publish it.

The *Tobin* trial

Two years later, on June 6, 2001, another trial, *Tobin vs SmithKline Beecham*, began in the District Court in Cheyenne, Wyoming.

Don Schell, an oilman who had had two brief episodes of nervous problems lasting a matter of a week or two in the 80s, when feeling nervous in 1990 had been put on Prozac by his doctor. On Prozac, he became agitated and had possibly begun to hear voices before discontinuing it, after which he improved. For the next eight years, he had no further nervous problems. Then in 1998, a spell of anxiety with some sleep disturbance took him to his family doctor for a sleeping pill. He was given a sleeping pill plus Paxil, with the doctor recording his problems as anxiety and insomnia—neither of which triggers homicide or suicide. His daughter Deborah was visiting for the weekend with the Schells' only grandchild, nine-month-old Alyssa. Forty-eight hours after starting Paxil, Schell put three bullets through the head of his wife Rita, three bullets through Deborah's head and three through Alyssa's head before killing himself. His son-in-law Tim Tobin brought a case against SmithKline.

The experts for Tim Tobin were Terry Maltsberger and David Healy. Maltsberger made a convincing case that Schell's behavior could only be explained in terms of a drug-induced delirium. Healy brought SmithKline's healthy volunteer trials into play. In these trials done in completely healthy people, many volunteers had suffered agitation and depression in addition to withdrawal symptoms after taking Paxil for just a couple of weeks. In some trials up to 85% of the volunteers who had been on this drug for only two or three weeks had demonstrated withdrawal problems when they halted. Among these healthy volunteers was one who had committed suicide and several who became aggressive.

During the trial Ian Hudson, who had just changed jobs from worldwide safety director for SmithKline to Director of Licensing for Britain's regulatory agency, stated that in an individual case, one cannot tell whether a drug is responsible for a violent or suicidal act—only randomized controlled trials can do that. Only after trials conclusively show a drug can cause suicide can it be said in any individual case that the drug might have caused suicide.

The jury members didn't agree. They figured there was no way to explain what happened other than to invoke Paxil's effects. The court ruled that SmithKline was 80% responsible for the deaths for failure to provide doctors with pertinent information and warnings and awarded $6.4 million to Tim Tobin[43]. In the same week as the *Tobin* verdict, in June 2001, a judge in Sydney, Australia, accepted the case put forward by both the defense and prosecution that but for his exposure to Zoloft, David Hawkins would not have killed his wife.

When the regulatory agency, the MHRA[44], later promoted Ian Hudson to Chief Executive, Healy stated, "If he takes the position with the MHRA that he took at the trial, then none of us is safe with any drug in the U.K. at the moment. How would Mr. Hudson even be able to blame alcohol for making someone drunk?"

After the *Tobin* verdict on June 25, 2001, SmithKline complied with a request from the British regulator to issue a warning to doctors and to patients about paroxetine, at the same time insisting the timing of the warning had nothing to do with the *Tobin* decision.

The warning read, "The possibility of suicide is inherent in depression and may persist until significant therapeutic effect is achieved, and it is general clinical experience with all antidepressant therapies that the risk of suicide may increase in the early stages of recovery." The problem with this wording is that the person taking the drug is left thinking he or she has a problem, rather than that the pill can cause the problem.

In December 2001, the Drug Safety Committee of the MHRA reviewed the suicidal behaviour, aggression and akathisia issue, concluding that the possibility of this affecting "a small high-risk population could not be ruled out." It advised adding the risk of akathisia to all SSRI Summaries of Product Characteristics (SPC). The assessment report was discussed at a European

PharmacoVigilance Working Party meeting, which agreed, but considered that further discussion was required to clarify the definition of the term *akathisia*.

Following *Tobin*, GlaxoSmithKline (GSK) faced a series of suicide cases as well as class actions for dependence on Paxil. These were settled out of court. As Bloomberg put it:[45]

> *The London-based company hasn't disclosed the settlement total in company filings. It has made public some accords. Glaxo's provision for legal and other non-tax disputes as of the end of 2008 was 1.9 billion pounds ($3.09 billion), according to its latest annual report. This included all legal matters, not just Paxil... About 450 suicide-related Paxil cases were settled. Only about a dozen haven't been, the [Glaxo spokespeople] said.*

The importance of these lawsuits was not the money but the documents that came into the public domain. These contributed to a later Department of Justice action against GSK.

Much later, on October 13, 2009, GSK lost a Paxil-induced birth defect case, *Kilker vs GlaxoSmithKline*, and was ordered to pay $2.5 million. This verdict led to a further series of settlements involving more than 600 claims totaling significantly over $1 billion. Bloomberg reported on the verdict as follows:

> *GlaxoSmithKline Plc must pay $2.5 million over claims that its Paxil antidepressant caused birth defects, a Pennsylvania jury concluded in the first of 600 such cases to come to trial.*
>
> *Jurors in state court in Philadelphia deliberated about seven hours over two days before finding Glaxo failed to properly warn doctors and pregnant users of Paxil's risk. The panel awarded $2.5 million in compensatory damages to the family of Lyam Kilker. The 3-year-old was born with heart defects his mother blamed on the drug...*
>
> *It's the first time a jury has considered claims that Glaxo, the U.K.'s largest drugmaker, knew Paxil caused birth defects and hid the risk to*

> *increase profits... "The company disagrees with the verdict and will appeal," Kevin Colgan, a spokesman, said in an e-mailed statement.*
>
> *"While we sympathize with Lyam Kilker and his family, the scientific evidence does not establish that exposure to Paxil during pregnancy caused his condition," Colgan said.*

But for the most part, the world knew nothing about these verdicts. GSK, Lilly and Pfizer are adept at shutting down bad news. Clinicians to this day believe there is no risk of suicide from antidepressants, no risk of homicide, no risk of birth defects or of autistic spectrum disorder (ASD), no risk of alcoholism, no risk of permanent sexual dysfunction (PSSD), even though the labels of these drugs have quietly conceded these risks for some time.

In the U.K., Sarah Boseley from *The Guardian* began writing about Prozac with the *Forsyth* trial in 1999. Her articles cut closer and closer to the bone as there was no pushback from Lilly, or from GlaxoSmithKline when she began tackling Seroxat, as Paxil is known in the U.K. Altogether she wrote 60 articles on one aspect or another of the issues related to the SSRIs—from hidden risks to ghostwriting of reports. But there was little response from organized medicine—or anyone else.

Note: Interviews cited in Chapters 3-5 are available on Study329.org

CHAPTER 6

The Secrets of Study 329

The story of Study 329 began in Pennsylvania, ten years before Shelley Jofre flew there.

In 1992, Neil Ryan from the Department of Child Psychiatry at the University of Pittsburgh drew up a protocol for a trial of antidepressants in children. Few child psychiatrists at the time had many dealings with pharmaceutical companies, so he contacted Marty Keller, the Chair of Psychiatry at Brown University in Providence, Rhode Island. Others involved included Boris Birmaher, also from Pittsburgh, Michael Strober from UCLA, and Rachel Klein from Cohen Children's Medical Centre in New York.

The trial aimed to test an SSRI against imipramine and placebo for adolescent depression. Keller suggested approaching SmithKline Beecham (SB), whose Paxil had just been licensed for the treatment of depression in adults. It was standard at the time when a drug was approved for FDA to encourage companies to study the drug in children to establish its profile. SmithKline embraced the idea and adopted the trial design that Ryan, Keller and colleagues brought with them. The trial became known as Study 329.

Recruitment began in 1994, initially with Barbara Geller from Renard Hospital at Washington University in St. Louis; Marty Keller at Brown; Harold Koplewicz and Rachel Klein at Cohen Children's Medical Centre in New York; Stan Kutcher from Sunnybrook Health Science Centre in Toronto; Neal Ryan and Boris Birmaher at the Western Psychiatric Institute and Clinic in Pittsburgh; and Michael Strober and Robbie Wong from UCLA Medical Center in Los Angeles. Because recruitment was slow, the study was later expanded to include 10 centres in the United States and two in Canada.

Giving antidepressants to children was then an issue full of ambiguities. In the United States, where Freudian thinking had been dominant, the view had been that because the superego didn't appear until a later developmental stage, children were incapable of getting depressed. In Europe, there were no presumptions that children couldn't get depressed—there was simply the observation that they never got melancholia. They certainly could be miserable and unhappy, but the assumption was that this misery and unhappiness stemmed from their circumstances. The standard view was that support from an understanding adult would usually be all that was needed to overcome the problems.

This said, Verbena Kuhn, wife of Roland Kuhn who discovered the antidepressant effects of imipramine, had given it to children for "depression" in the 1960s.[46] Imipramine was widely given in the 1960s in low doses as a treatment for enuresis, seen by some as a behavioural issue. In fact, it's norepinephrine reuptake inhibiting properties can cause urinary retention in the exact same way as Cymbalta's similar action causes "bladder stabilization".

Imipramine had also been given by Rachel and Don Klein to their four-year old daughter who was intensely anxious and having panic episodes.[47] In a 1962 trial with patients in Hillside Hospital in New York, Klein and Max Fink had shown that imipramine and chlorpromazine were equally effective for depression but that imipramine was distinctly better for certain forms of anxiety. Chasing this lead, Klein came up with the concept of panic disorder and proposed imipramine as a specific treatment for this—and gave it to his daughter.

Following the launch of the SSRIs, by the mid-1990s, there were close to 70 open trials of SSRIs in children with almost all reporting benefits. The problem was that 15 randomized clinical trials (RCTs) of the tricyclic antidepressants had returned negative results—there was no positive trial. Ryan and his group hoped the SSRIs could be shown to work in RCTs in children where the older antidepressants hadn't. But the first paediatric RCT of Prozac, reporting in 1990, was also negative.

Could the SSRIs, which marketing portrayed as cleaner and safer than the older drugs, be shown to work for children with the right trial design? Having run a trial of imipramine some years earlier that failed, Kim Puig-Antich, also from Pittsburgh, had designed a Childhood Depression Scale—the Kiddie SADs. This would be used in Study 329 in the hope that it would be more sensitive than the standard depression rating scale—the Hamilton Depression Rating Scale. The HDRS, also called the HAM-D, had been designed in 1960 for trials of imipramine in adult melancholia. Perhaps the problem in children's trials was a rating scale one.

The design pitted Paxil against imipramine and placebo. Imipramine is also a serotonin reuptake inhibiting drug, among other things, but earlier trials had suggested it wouldn't work. The protocol proposed using imipramine in doses of up to 300 mg, which was double or triple the dose used for adults in clinical practice. Against this dose, there was every chance at the very least that the side-effect profile of Paxil would look good.

In adults, antidepressants had typically been tested in six-week trials. This is called the acute phase. Some trials were extended to eight weeks if it was thought the treatment might not work quickly. Study 329 opted for an eight-week duration in case the issue with children was a delayed response.

Study 329 also had a continuation phase. There were no data on giving antidepressants to children for longer than 8 weeks. Extending the trial for a further six months after the end of the acute phase offered a chance to see whether any useful effects might be picked up during that period.

The first child entered the study on April 20, 1994. The last child entered on March 20, 1997. Given that a six-month continuation phase still had to run, the very last measurements took place in early 1998.

As recruitment to Study 329 was slow, in April 1995 SmithKline began a further trial, Study 377, comparing Paxil and placebo in childhood depression, run out of 33 centres in Belgium, Italy, Spain, Britain, Holland, Canada, South Africa, United Arab Emirates, Argentina and Mexico. This was exactly the kind of scenario *Panorama*'s Ed Harriman saw coming. In the mid-1990s,

"Third World" countries were emerging as sites for clinical trials. They had research subjects who were drug-naive and possibly more inclined to participate in order to get the benefits of Western medication when they were unable to get any treatment in their home setting.

Parallel to these SmithKline studies, Lilly was running trials of Prozac. There was also a study of citalopram in Europe organised by Lundbeck. The recruitment for this was very slow as European clinicians found cases of depression to be even rarer than in the United States. Pfizer was also running studies on Zoloft for OCD and depression. Karen Wagner, one of the Study 329 authors, ended up as the lead author on Pfizer's depression studies and on a later Forest study of citalopram.

In early 1997, on behalf of the British Association for Psychopharmacology, David Healy convened a workshop on psychotropic drug use in children.[48] The backdrop was that there were difficulties giving any psychotropic drugs to children in Britain, even though it was clear in some instances stimulants could help some children with ADHD and also that antidepressants, and in particular SSRIs, could help some cases of obsessive-compulsive disorder. It was Healy's involvement with this workshop that led to a later approach from Shelley Jofre when *Panorama*, BBC-TV's flagship investigative journalism program, a few years later decided to investigate the rapidly growing use of stimulants for ADHD in Britain.

The speakers at this workshop included Stan Kutcher and Rachel Klein, who told everyone that a Prozac study by Graham Emslie was on its way to publication and would give a positive finding for Prozac. This would be a breakthrough in efforts to demonstrate that SSRIs could be helpful for depressed children. They also made it clear they were involved in a Paxil study in children who were depressed. They gave no more details, other than to say this would give the first-ever data on benefits of an SSRI over an extended period of time.

The Emslie study was published at the end of 1997.[49] While the article claims Prozac had been shown to work, FDA medical and statistical reviews of the study undertaken when Lilly submitted this and a later study as part of its application for a licence for Prozac to treat depressed children make clear the trial was negative. The FDA ultimately approved Prozac, but technically speaking this and a later Prozac trial were failed trials. The Emslie study, when it was published, was sold as hugely positive; no one had access to the data showing a reality at odds with the publication and the hoopla.

By the time Study 329 finished in early 1998, the stakes were higher than they had been when the study began. In 1997, an amendment to the FDA's Prescription Drug User Fee Act (PDUFA) offered six months of patent extension to companies that provided data on the use of their drug in children even if the drug hadn't been shown to work. At the time, Paxil was heading towards sales of $2 billion per annum and six months' patent extension was worth several hundred million dollars.

In 2001, Lilly submitted two negative Prozac trials to the FDA, where they found FDA not just willing to endorse patent extension but also to approve the drug for use in children. The Paxil trials had the same format as the Prozac trials, with many of the same investigators.

On January 1, 2001, SmithKline Beecham and Glaxo Wellcome merged to become GlaxoSmithKline (GSK), then the biggest pharmaceutical company in the world. In July 2001, the Keller et al glowingly positive publication of the results of Study 329 appeared. In early 2002, GSK opened negotiations with the FDA on a license application to claim Paxil could treat depressed children. In August, the final submission of their paediatric trials in anxiety and depression, of which three dealt with depression, Studies 329, 377 and 701, was sent to FDA. FDA then had eight weeks under the new PDUFA arrangements to announce whether it was likely to approve the drug or not.

Is there a story here?

After the GSK merger, *Panorama*, BBC TV's flagship investigative journalism programme, began considering the possibility of a programme focusing on GSK, which was based a few miles away from the BBC's headquarters in

Britain. And in June 2001, almost coincident with the publication of Study 329, a jury in Cheyenne, Wyoming, returned a verdict in *Tobin vs SmithKline* against GSK for Paxil-induced homicide and suicide, a first-ever verdict against a pharmaceutical company for a behavioural effect of its drug. Healy was one of the experts for the plaintiff and was based in the U.K.

In early 2001, Healy had managed to attract attention for another reason.[50] In 2000, he had been recruited to the University of Toronto and was due to move there in April 2001. He had also been approached to be an expert in the *Tobin* case. In July 2000, during a meeting in the U.K., one of the guest lecturers, Charlie Nemeroff, had approached Healy and told him that he, Nemeroff, was due to be an expert on the opposite side. Work Healy had been doing on suicidality on antidepressants, Nemeroff said, would cost Healy his career.

Nemeroff had moved up in the world since 1991 when he presented the data supposedly exonerating Prozac from a risk of suicide at the FDA hearings on the issue. He had become the Head of the Psychiatry Department at Emory University in Atlanta. He featured on the front cover of the September 2000 issue of The Economics of Neuroscience with a strapline "Boss of Bosses. Is the brash and controversial Charles Nemeroff the most powerful man in psychiatry?" It later transpired that he was pulling in around $1 million per year at the time in consulting fees from GSK alone.

Healy and Nemeroff were both on the programme for a meeting in Toronto at the end of November 2000 to celebrate the 75th anniversary of the University of Toronto's Department of Psychiatry and the 150th anniversary of Mental Health Services on Queen Street. There was an international cast of speakers. Healy's talk outlined the contents of The Creation of Psychopharmacology, a book about the history of antipsychotics scheduled for publication by Harvard University Press. Healy's was the highest-rated talk of the meeting, Nemeroff's the lowest-rated.

During the meeting, Nemeroff had words with senior people at the University of Toronto who had been involved in hiring Healy a few months beforehand and told them they didn't want to go through with the appointment—Healy should be let go. A key person Nemeroff talked to was David Goldbloom, on whom he apparently had quite an impact. Goldbloom attempted to get hold of Healy over the next few days, but Healy had flown to New York. Nemeroff had also gone to an American Foundation for Suicide Prevention meeting in New York and was telling people there the following day that Healy had lost his job at the University of Toronto. Healy gave several talks in New York in different settings over the following few days, repeating the Toronto talk in one, which was as well received as it had been in Toronto. He then received an email from Goldbloom telling him that his talk had been "problematic," and that he was fired.

The story came to light in April 2001 because Healy, figuring the first question on the witness stand in the *Tobin* case would be, "Isn't it true doctor that you were recently fired by the University of Toronto?", decided that the only way to pre-empt this was to go public. He did so with help from Sarah Boseley of *The Guardian*. GSK filed a motion with the court to ensure there would be no mention of the Toronto affair in court.

All of this interested *Panorama*. Shelley Jofre was picked to be the "lips" on what would be "The Secrets of Seroxat". She touched base with Healy, and then headed to the American Psychiatric Association meeting in Philadelphia in May 2002.

She was handed Study 329 to read by Harriman on the plane. Harriman's plan was to expose the fact that trials like this were exploiting children from deprived communities—which they had done in the case of Study 377. But the interviewees in the case of Study 329 didn't show any sensitivity on this point. Then Neal Ryan grew visibly uncomfortable at being questioned about the term emotional lability in the paper.

Uncertain about what she was dealing with, Jofre followed up her interview with Ryan with an email to get him to clarify what he'd said to her. Meanwhile, Ryan contacted GSK saying a journalist had been in touch with him and could they advise on how best to respond.

Emotional lability

The issue of emotional lability had just come onto the FDA's radar from another source as well. Just after GSK submitted its application for the approval of Paxil for paediatric use, on August 28, two plaintiffs' lawyers, Don Farber and Skip Murgatroyd, then prosecuting Paxil adult cases, met with FDA's Steve Galson, Deputy Director of Drug Evaluation and Research, and told him that GSK had been coding suicidal events as "emotional lability."

Six weeks later, on October 7, 2002, the front cover of *Newsweek* in the United States featured an unhappy teenage girl and a strapline "Teen Depression: 3 Million Kids Suffer From It. What You Can Do." The message was that depression would cost children their careers, their relationships, their lives, and if not treated would lead to alcohol and drug abuse and other problems. The answer to all this was that Prozac had just been approved for the treatment of children, and Paxil and Zoloft were about to be approved.

On October 10, World Mental Health Day, and the 40th anniversary of the signing of the 1962 amendments to the *FDA Act*, the FDA sent a letter to GlaxoSmithKline which stated, "We have completed the review of this application and it is approvable." [51]

In addition, as is standard with approvable letters, the FDA asked for further details on a series of items, 12 all told, including:

> *7. [You] have listed paroxetine treated patients who experienced adverse events coded under the terms hostility, emotional lability or agitation. However the table did not include placebo patients nor did it include psychiatric adverse events that were coded under other terms. Please prepare an expanded version of this table including all psychiatric and behavioral adverse events and also those that occur among placebo patients. In addition it would be helpful if you could attach the narrative case summaries for those events that were either serious or resulted in premature discontinuation.*
>
> *8. Please provide your rationale for coding suicide attempts and other forms of self-injurious behavior under the term emotional lability.*

On October 13, *Panorama*'s "The Secrets of Seroxat" aired in Britain.[52] The program covered suicidality on paroxetine, dependence and addiction to paroxetine, and the testing of the drug on children. Among the highlights was a set-piece between Jofre and Alastair Benbow, the head of European clinical psychiatry for GSK. Jofre's approach was shaped by the fact that she was now certain that many emotional lability events involved suicidality. She put this to Benbow, who in response stated,

> *There are a number of allegations that you made there, none of which are correct... In terms of whether we think Seroxat should be made available to children? Absolutely. Two percent of children, four percent of adolescents would develop depression. The adolescents are at particular risk of suicide. Suicide in adolescents is the third leading cause of death. The vast majority of these patients did not have side effects significant enough to withdraw from treatment. The reality is that in this population depression is an extremely serious condition and in many cases leads to suicide.*

In response to this program, *Panorama* had 65,000 calls and more than 1,300 emails—the greatest response they had ever had to any program up to then. The responses endorsed what the program had reported—that paroxetine was linked to suicidality and dependence. *Panorama* had never repeated a topic before but ultimately made three more programs on GSK and paroxetine.

Turmoil in GSK

These calls and emails laid the basis for the second program on the topic. *Panorama* handed the production reins over to Andy Bell, a veteran of the Northern Irish troubles. The second program, "Emails from the Edge,"[53] aired on May 11, 2003. For this episode, Jofre again interviewed Alastair Benbow, who on this occasion said,

> *The safety profile in children is very similar to that in adults, with a couple of exceptions, and we have provided that updated safety information to regulatory authorities around the world and specifically in relation*

> *to the potential for an increase in suicidal thoughts or suicidal attempts... This increase is small. It is rather similar to, if you imagine a school of more than a thousand children, all of whom are deeply troubled by depression, less than a small class size would have these suicidal thoughts or attempts.*

The screening of "Emails from the Edge" led the leading patient advocate group for mental health issues in the United Kingdom, MIND, to protest outside the building of Britain's drug regulator, the MHRA, in London. The MHRA announced a reactivation of an Expert Working Group that had been looking at the issues of suicide and dependence on SSRIs. First set up in 2002, this had been disbanded because of undeclared conflicts of interest.

GSK was under intense pressure. In May, coincident with "Emails from the Edge", the company produced a glossy brochure internally for staff, one of several brochures and advertisements under the heading of "Science with a Conscience" prepared at this time.

PAGE 1 - BROCHURE COVER:

> HEADLINE: ***Were the UK doctors who wrote 4,580,000 prescriptions for Seroxat last year right?***

PAGE 2 - INSIDE LEFT :

> HEADLINE: ***If you are depressed who should you consult? A TV presenter or a doctor?***
>
> COPY: *Seroxat has helped tens of millions of people lead fuller and more productive lives.*
>
> *At GlaxoSmithKline we believe that the best people for patients to consult about their treatment are their own doctors. Who knows more about the background of each individual patient and the appropriate treatment for different conditions?*

Unlike TV reporters doctors are aware of the huge advances that have been made in the treatment of depression in the last few years. Seroxat is an SSRI, a breakthrough in the treatment of depression and anxiety.

As a class, SSRI's are probably some of the most extensively investigated medicines available in the UK today.

Their safety is constantly monitored by the Medicines and Healthcare Products Regulatory Agency (MHRA)—a rather more expert body than the producers of Panorama.

PAGE 3 – INSIDE RIGHT

HEADLINE: ***Depression affects 5 million people in the UK. Seroxat is a highly effective answer.***

COPY: *Seroxat is an effective treatment with a well established safety profile and a wealth of positive experience involving thousands of doctors, tens of millions of patients and over ten years experience worldwide since its UK launch in 1991.*

Seroxat is not addictive.

Seroxat prevents suicide by treating depression and helping to reduce suicidal thoughts.

The majority of patients do not get side effects on either taking Seroxat or stopping.

We have total faith in Seroxat so can you.

By 2020 the World Health Organisation estimates that depression will be the second most burdensome illness worldwide. Depression is a potentially deadly disease that affects a huge number of people in the UK.

At any one time 1 in 7 people are affected by depression. Worse still 1 in 7 people with depression commit suicide. Every year this results in the death of 3,000 people in the UK with devastating consequences for their friends and family.

However there is good news. As antidepressant usage has increased suicide rates have fallen at 15% during the 1990's.

PAGE 4 - BACK COVER:

HEADLINE: ***Judge Seroxat on clinical trials not trial by media.***

COPY: *Contrary to the claims of the* Panorama *programme:*

- *In clinical trials of over 9,000 patients treated with Seroxat, the majority of the reporting symptoms on stopping were short lived, mild to moderate in intensity and the majority resolved on their own within two weeks.*
- *There is no compelling evidence that Seroxat is linked to an increased risk of suicide.*
- *Data shows that Seroxat will reduce violence and aggression and help prevent self harm.*

We take every single report seriously. No treatment is perfect for every individual patient and it is up to the doctor to decide in conjunction with the patient exactly what treatment is best for them. And bear in mind in clinical trials, 60% of patients who took the placebo experienced side effects that they thought were related to the treatment.

At almost exactly the same time as this brochure was produced, in a letter dated May 22, 2003, GSK wrote to Russell Katz of the FDA and other regulators to update them—as Alistair Benbow several weeks earlier on *Panorama* had claimed they had already done—on the safety issues in children linked to Paxil-Seroxat.[54]

The contents of GSK's May 22 letter to the FDA were at odds with the brochure produced for internal company consumption. The submissions to FDA showed that Paxil-Seroxat doubled the rate of suicidal acts in children and did so in a statistically significant way compared to placebo. It showed an increased risk of suicidality during the active phase and 30-day taper phase in both Study 329 on its own and in GSK's trials on children in general.

Where the internal GSK material had stated there was no evidence linking paroxetine to violence, material presented to an MHRA working group around this time showed a doubling of violent acts on paroxetine compared to placebo.

Where the internal GSK material denied any risk of addiction or dependence, the material presented to the MHRA showed Symptoms on Stopping in a majority of healthy volunteers after exposures as short as two weeks.

Shortly after this, Healy was contacted by Rose Firestein from the office of New York's Attorney General, Elliot Spitzer. What could he tell her about GSK's trials in children? His answer was the Paxil trials didn't show it worked but did show it caused problems. He gave her the protocol numbers and suggested she apply to GSK for the Clinical Study Reports, and if they came she should look closely at things like emotional lability.

Next steps

Ten days after GSK's letter to FDA's director for CNS drugs, Russell Katz, on June 2, Katz sent an email to Andrew Mosholder, one of the original reviewers of the Paxil dossier that had led to the approvable letter, stating,

> *Andy—Hi, hope you are well.*
>
> *We have recently become aware of a presumed association between paroxetine and suicidality in paediatric patients. We received a call from the EMEA a little over a week ago. Dr Raines told us that the company [GSK] had submitted data that demonstrated that use of paroxetine in kids was associated with increased suicidality compared to placebo, and that the company proposed labelling changes. I believe she also said that it was in the news, and that it was a big issue. Tom [Laughren] and I told her that the company had not informed us of any of this and we agreed to look into it.*[55]

This was after GSK had sent Katz their letter explaining exactly these points. As Katz's email hints, MHRA, for which Dr. June Raine worked, was faced with patient groups protesting outside its building. This and the internal brochure the company had felt obliged to produce to reassure its own staff indicates the level of disquiet after the *Panorama* program.

On June 10, the MHRA acted to contraindicate paroxetine and other SSRIs in children and adolescents.

GSK then issued a series of *Dear Doctor* letters which made it clear that paroxetine should not be given to children who are depressed and that there was an increased risk of problems linked to agitation and suicidality both on treatment and on withdrawal from treatment.

At the end of June, the FDA also issued an advisory noting concern about prescribing antidepressants in children.

Around this time, Andy Bell was sent a tranche of GSK documents that an employee had accidentally left behind on a photocopying machine. These outlined GSK's marketing plans for Seroxat-Paxil during the 2001 and 2002 period, aimed at making it the best-selling antidepressant in the world. There were position papers detailing its strengths and weaknesses vis-à-vis other antidepressants. Some of these provided source material for Christopher Lane's book on the marketing of social anxiety disorder, *Shyness: How Normal Behavior Became a Sickness,*[56] which came out some years later.

Bell also found a brown envelope in his office mailbox one day. This contained another document that shaped everything from that point onwards. He took it to the BBC bosses who had figured two *Panorama* shows on Paxil were enough. A third was inconceivable.

The genesis of a scientific fact

Despite the FDA's advisory and despite being in receipt of a later analysis from GSK making it clear that paroxetine caused adolescents to become suicidal, and despite SSRIs being discouraged in Europe, senior FDA officers began to downplay the risks. On October 28, the *New York Times* and *Washington Post* reported the agency as less convinced there was a problem. They were analyzing the data prior to a full Pediatric Psychopharmacological Drugs Advisory Committee (PDAC) meeting scheduled for February 2, 2004.

At the end of January 2004, days before the PDAC meeting on antidepressants and suicide, an American College of Neuropsychopharmacology (ACNP) working group, which included a number of the authors of Study 329, issued a position paper stating that there was no problem with antidepressants and suicide. ACNP at this point still had a good reputation in the academic community. This paper got widespread national coverage.[57] Achieving such coverage had been part of the deal offered by GYMR, the public relations agency Get Your Message Right that had in fact written the ACNP report.

On February 1, the *San Francisco Chronicle* broke a story claiming that FDA's reviewer on the suicide issue, Andy Mosholder, had been gagged. Mosholder was the internal FDA reviewer whom Katz had approached in June 2003 to look at the issue of emotional lability in greater depth. When he reported that there was a statistically significant doubling of the risk of suicidal acts by children on antidepressants, FDA would not allow him to share his findings at the February 2 meeting.

The February 2 meeting appeared to be geared up to clearing the use of SSRIs in children. At midday on February 2, at a press conference midway through the proceedings, Bell released his brown envelope document. This six-page document had a cover note by Jackie Westaway with distribution to senior marketing and medical personnel within GSK. It had been prepared in October 1998:

> *Please find attached to this memo a position piece, prepared by Julie Wilson of CMAT, summarizing the results of the clinical studies in adolescent depression.*
>
> *As you well know the results of the studies were disappointing in that we did not reach statistical significance on the primary end points and thus the data do not support a label claim for the treatment of adolescent depression. The possibility of obtaining a safety statement from this data was considered but rejected. The best which could have been achieved*

was a statement that although safety data was reassuring, efficacy had not been demonstrated. Consultation of the marketing teams via Regulatory confirmed that this would be unacceptable commercially.[58]

The document from CMAT, SmithKline's Central Medical Affairs Team, "Seroxat/Paxil Position Piece on the Phase III Clinical Studies 329 and 377," includes the following statements:

> *Conclusions from these studies:*
>
> - *There were no differences in the safety profile of Seroxat/Paxil in adolescents when compared to that already established in the adult population.*
> - *The efficacy data from the above clinical trials are insufficiently robust to support a regulatory submission and label change for this patient population.*
> - *Based on the current data, and following consultation with SB country regulatory and marketing groups, no regulatory submission will be made for either efficacy of safety statements relating to adolescent depression… [because]:*
> - *regulatory agencies would not approve a statement indicating that there are no safety issues in adolescents, as this could be seen as promoting off-label use.*
> - *It would be commercially unacceptable to include a statement that efficacy had not been demonstrated, as this would undermine the profile of paroxetine.*
>
> ***Target:*** *To effectively manage the dissemination of these data in order to minimise any potentially negative commercial impact.*
>
> ***Proposals:*** *Positive data from Study 329 will be published in abstract form… and a full manuscript of the 329 data will be progressed.*

In 2001, the "positive data" became the Keller et al. *JAACAP* article.

GSK's immediate response to the document was to claim that it had been prepared by a consultancy agency. It in no way reflected the position of the company. They made this claim even though the approvable letter from FDA in October 2002 had noted,

> *We agree that the results of Study 329 failed to demonstrate the efficacy of Paroxetine in paediatric patients with MDD. Given the fact that negative trials are frequently seen even for antidepressant drugs that we know are effective, we agree that it would not be useful to describe these negative trials in the labelling.*

At the February 2 PDAC meeting, Bob Temple and Russell Katz denied point blank that there had been any contact between FDA and other regulatory agencies. Later, evidence such as Katz's email to Mosholder outlining his phone call with June Raine of the MHRA suggests regulators lie pretty easily.

The advisory committee on February 2 indicated that there were grounds for concern that antidepressants did cause some minors to become suicidal and little evidence that they worked. [59]But rather than take action, FDA proposed an adjournment while a Columbia University working group reviewed all the behavioural events in these trials to work out a rigorous classification system that would allow all parties to agree on the data to be included and excluded. The hearings would reconvene on September 13 and 14.

There was no obvious scientific rationale for this manoeuvre but it had been planned before the PDAC hearing took place.

The good wife

The next step unfolded on March 2. One of the people who picked up Andy Bell's brown envelope document was linked to the *Canadian Medical Association Journal* (CMAJ). She asked Healy if it was okay to publish this and then did so as part of a piece entitled "Drug Company Experts Advised Staff to Withhold Data About SSRI Use in Children." It begins,

> *An internal document advised staff at the international drug giant GlaxoSmithKline (GSK) to withhold clinical trial findings in 1998 that indicated the antidepressant paroxetine (Paxil in North America and Seroxat in the UK) had no beneficial effect in treating adolescents.*[60]

The *CMAJ* article was linked to the CMAT document. This brought it to the attention of Rose Firestein in the Office of the Attorney General in New York. The acknowledgement that Study 329 was a negative study but that the good bits would be selected from it and published provided the key piece of evidence in support of a lawsuit against GSK for fraud.

On March 10, Congressmen Joe Barton (R-Texas) and Jim Greenwood (R-Pennsylvania) stated that they planned to launch an investigation of FDA's handling of the SSRI issue in children. Senator Grassley's office did the same. Emilia di Santo and Michelle Andersen from Grassley's office were contacted by an FDA employee, most likely David Graham, one of FDA's lead safety officers.

One of the little-known aspects of this story is that Graham and Mosholder, and some others in FDA were committed Christians, who were rather wary of the State, believing in home-schooling their children for instance.

On March 19, Andersen contacted the FDA. After her call, the FDA convened a press conference with one hour's notice. At the conference the FDA informed the media that the FDA was issuing an advisory to all companies requiring a warning on antidepressants.

The warning denied a causal link had been established, but it linked warnings to starting and stopping treatment and to dose changes and to the use of SSRIs for everything from obsessive-compulsive disorders and smoking to depression. This warning means "caused".

In April, an editorial in *The Lancet*, titled "Depressing Research,"[61] deplored the situation in which researchers had been fooled into thinking that antidepressants worked for children when the data showed just the opposite. The editorial called this a crisis for evidence-based medicine. But Boris Birmaher in *JAACAP* (which published the Keller paper), Bernard Vitiello in the *New*

England Journal of Medicine and Harold Koplewicz in the *Journal of Child and Adolescent Psychopharmacology* claimed the fuss was deterring patients from seeking treatment and would cost lives. Birmaher and Koplewicz were both authors on Study 329.

A few weeks later, on June 3, New York State Attorney General Eliot Spitzer filed a fraud action in New York State Supreme Court accusing British drug giant GlaxoSmithKline PLC of "repeated and persistent fraud" for concealing known problems with efficacy and safety of Paxil (paroxetine) for children and adolescents. The suit argued that GSK hid the fact that in some of its trials Paxil failed to show better efficacy in adolescents and children than a placebo and in some cases could be more likely to cause suicidal thinking.

A charge of consumer fraud for medication was unprecedented. There was a good basis for the charge, given that Study 329 and other GSK trials in paediatric groups may represent the greatest divide in all of medicine between what the academic literature says about the drugs and what the data actually show. The key element however was the CMAT document, which offered evidence of an intent to deceive.

Spitzer held a press conference at which he claimed his office's action would change the course of medicine for ever. All pharmaceutical companies would be pressured into making their data available to doctors—as it should be.

That same week *The Lancet* called on GSK to publish all its trial data, and on June 10, GSK posted executive summaries of its paediatric clinical trials on the company website.

Meanwhile at the end of June, the Columbia group under Kelly Posner submitted its completed review to the FDA. All the indications are that this had been intended to make the problem go away, but the problems were multiplying.

On August 26, just three weeks before the next PDAC hearing, GSK announced that it would pay US$2.5 million as part of a settlement of the Spitzer lawsuit. It also agreed to publicly disclose all of its clinical trials about the safety of paroxetine for children in a "Clinical Trials Registry."

But showing a mastery of the art of turning problems into opportunities, the company's press release said:

> *"We are pleased that the Attorney General believes the Clinical Trial Register we have been developing will provide useful information to the medical and scientific community," said Mark Werner, Senior Vice President for U.S. Legal Operations at GlaxoSmithKline. "We believe that GlaxoSmithKline's initiative to launch this register is a responsible step in ensuring transparency of our clinical trial data."*[62]

Spitzer was furious.

This was the latest in a series of high profile cases against financial corruption on Wall Street that had underpinned speculation he was using these cases to underpin a run for Governor. His apparently successful action to rein in the pharmaceutical industry strengthened his reputation. In 2006, he became Governor.

But in 2008, he was forced to resign after being found in a compromising escort situation. The first season of the television serial *The Good Wife* and the last episode of *Law and Order* are widely thought to have drawn from the Spitzer story, including the details of his compromising. There was no end of speculation as to who had been behind the downfall.

It is difficult to believe the resolution of the New York case did not influence the September 14 PDAC Hearings. The Hearings may also have been influenced by Congressional Action to investigate the gagging of Andy Mosholder, which started on September 9. It was very clear that Mosholder was going to say that his disinterested reading of the results showed a problem but that officials higher in the system at FDA took a different view, and blocked him.

The Columbia tallying of the suicidal events, under Kelly Posner, that was made public was almost identical to Mosholder's earlier one.

On September 14 the PDAC committee voted 15-8 in favour of a class-wide Black Box Warning for suicide related to antidepressants in children and adolescents. Russell Katz stated that FDA accepted that antidepressants cause suicidal behaviour.

Taken on trust

Panorama wasn't finished. The document that arrived in a brown envelope in Andy Bell's office mailbox provided the basis for a fraud action against GSK and later a U.S. Department of Justice action that resulted in the then-largest fine in corporate history.

But GSK was a British company, and the document originated in Britain. What were British regulators doing about it?

As early as October 1, 2003, the Pharmacovigilance Group of the MHRA began to grapple with the issue of GSK's failure to advise the regulator on a timely basis about issues relating to safety and lack of efficacy of Paroxetine. Unlike what happened in the United States, GSK's failure to advise the MHRA about the lack of efficacy and dangers of paroxetine did not result in a prosecution. MHRA offered a number of reasons as to why not:

- Relevant EU legislation requires the reporting of adverse reactions occurring in the normal conditions of use. A clinical trial in relation to an unlicensed indication did not fall within "normal conditions of use."
- Although EU legislation also required adverse events to be reported in "post authorisation studies," these did not include studies on a product outside of its licensed indications.
- U.K. legislation did require adverse events during clinical trials to be reported, but this requirement applied only to clinical trials in the U.K., and a failure to do so did not constitute a criminal offence.
- Although 2002 U.K. legislation required a marketing authorization holder's Qualified Person to report any information relevant to the risk/benefit evaluation of a product, the MRHA received legal advice that the legislation was not sufficiently clear that this obligation applied to clinical trials outside a product's licensed indications.

The bosses of *Panorama* now realized a third program was inevitable. In "Taken on Trust,"[63] Jofre confronted Alasdair Breckenridge, the head of Britain's MHRA. Breckenridge came out of the encounter badly, mumbling about explorations of a legal action against GSK when ultimately the MHRA and Britain did nothing. Breckenridge stepped aside soon after, being replaced by Kent Wood, who in turn has been replaced by Ian Hudson, formerly of GSK.

Ultimately MHRA and the British Government did nothing. GSK was a flagship British company.

Spin that no amount of data can overcome

On January 29, 2007, *Panorama* broadcast "Secrets of the Drug Trials."[64] In the last of four programs on paroxetine, Jofre explored the making of Study 329. The CMAT document had opened up a rich vein of exploration that Skip Murgatroyd from Baum Hedlund raised in depositions of Bob Temple and Paul Leber, leading figures within FDA during the period, as well as Sally Laden, Martin Keller, Neal Ryan and others.

It tells the story of how the facts about this drug were suppressed, even though they had been known to GSK and its predecessor companies from the outset. The episode shows how company officials promoted the drug for young people, knowing that it was neither effective nor safe. In this final program on the subject, Jofre asks *JAACAP* Editor Mina Dulcan a question:

> JOFRE: *Do you have any regrets about publishing this study?*
>
> DULCAN: *Oh, I don't have any regrets about publishing at all. It generated all sorts of useful discussion, which is the purpose of a scholarly journal.*

It transpired that SmithKline had approached Scientific Therapeutics International (STI) to write up Study 329. Sally Laden was given the brief. Laden was skilful at presenting Paxil in a favourable light. As James McCafferty, Laden's SmithKline contact, put it in a July 19, 1999, email:

> *It seems incongruous that we state that paroxetine [Paxil] is safe yet report so many SAEs [serious adverse events]. I know the investigators have not raised an issue, but I fear that the editors will. I am still not sure how to describe these events. I will again review all the SAEs to make myself feel comfortable about what we report in print.*

The article's appearance in the journal with the highest impact factor in the field, especially with an authorship line of 22 authors, including some of the biggest names in child psychiatry and psychopharmacology, claiming that the drug worked well and was safe, guaranteed a boost in sales of Paxil. Sales were particularly strong in New York, where several of the authors were based, and where the emergence of the CMAT document laid the basis for a fraud case.

This was the episode where Jofre got her chin stroked by Marty Keller.

The question for every reader is: How could a journalist with no medical training, Shelley Jofre, spot the problems that the authors and reviewers of Study 329 failed to detect?

Precisely because she was not in the field, the journal's reputation and the distinction of the names on the authorship line meant nothing to her. Because statistical significance was not part of her everyday world, she wasn't hypnotized into thinking that non-significant events weren't happening. She didn't assume "emotional lability" referred to some inconsequential change on treatment; she noticed that it was happening more on Paxil and began to ask questions. The lack of sensible answers ultimately led to the discovery of company documents conceding that Paxil didn't work and that the entire study was ghostwritten.

In 2016, we got fake news but as events were to reveal, medicine has been operating with fake science for thirty years. The trials we see bear as much relation to the data as what we get from politicians bears to the facts.

In contrast to what one imagines the position of the editor of the NYT might be had they published study 329, Mina Dulcan seems completely unfazed by her role in the publication of one of the most notorious studies of all time. At some point it is going to take a gutsy academic editor to risk being shut down by industry or the rest of us to consider whether we would be safer if clinical trials were published in the *New York Times* or *Panorama* with academic journals reclassified as periodicals and academic meetings as trade fairs.

But the lay media can only go so far. CBS' *60 Minutes* bottled out of having anything to do with the issue—having been handed a program about these issues on a plate even before *Panorama* aired its episodes. And *Panorama* later let Jofre go after she made one too many programs about GSK.

Note: Videos and transcripts cited in Chapter 6 are available on Study329.org

CHAPTER 7

Black Box, Black Arts

A sensational document leading to a successful fraud case that was going to change the face of medicine, a document that opened up the prospect of investigating ghost-writing, a Black Box Warning slapped on antidepressants after nearly 15 years of campaigning, might all sound good but it didn't feel at the time like much was really changing and it's not clear there has been any change for the better since.

Suicide might now seem to have been front and centre at the February PDAC meeting but actually there was a greater emphasis on whether the drugs had been shown to work. Even the internal GSK document that came into the frame talked about the efficacy of paroxetine rather than suicidality. There was a distance to travel before the SSRIs ended up with a Black Box Warning for suicide risk, and they may have only done so because there was no evidence of benefit from the drugs to put in the balance.

A Black Box Warning is the FDA's most explicit warning. It applies to drugs that may be beneficial but also have significant hazards—drugs that most physicians and patients would want to remain on the market but ideally accompanied by warnings. Few groups campaigning for warnings have wanted the SSRIs or other antidepressants to be removed from the market. The call has been for appropriate warnings.

Primed by Prozac

In 1992 when Paxil was approved, it was standard for the FDA to request studies of new medicines in children to assess efficacy and safety. Between 1992 and 2002, GSK ran nine clinical trials attempting to find evidence of efficacy in paroxetine for the treatment of depression and anxiety in paediatric populations. None of the trials demonstrated efficacy in mood disorders.

In 1997, the stakes rose when Congress passed the FDA Modernization Act (the FDAMA), and the Best Pharmaceuticals for Children Act (BPCA). These gave six-month patent extensions to drug makers who conducted paediatric clinical trials of existing drugs and submitted the data to the FDA, whether or not the drugs were effective. The stakes rose again when companies saw how the FDA dealt with Prozac for children.

In November 1997, Lilly published A Double-Blind, Randomized, *Placebo-Controlled Trial of Fluoxetine in Children and Adolescents with Depression.*[65] The first author, Graham Emslie, was also an author on Study 329. This was a trial of 96 youths, aged 7 to 17, with major depressive disorder. Emslie claimed that 27 out of 48 (56%) of those receiving fluoxetine (Prozac) and 16 out of 48 (33%) receiving placebo were rated "much" or "very much" improved. They concluded this showed that "fluoxetine was superior to placebo in the acute phase treatment of major depressive disorder in child and adolescent outpatients."

To get approval there needed to be a second study. The first study was funded by NIMH. The second, whose first author was also Emslie, was funded by Lilly. Both were submitted to FDA in 2000 as part of Lilly's application for approval to use Prozac in children and obtain the additional six-month patent exclusivity this would bring.

The second Emslie study was published in October 2002: "Fluoxetine for Acute Treatment of Depression in Children and Adolescents: A Placebo-Controlled, Randomized Clinical Trial".[66] In this study, 122 children and 97 adolescents with MDD were apparently randomly assigned to either placebo or fluoxetine. The authors reported that significantly more fluoxetine-treated patients (41%) met the prospectively defined criteria for remission than placebo-treated patients (20%). They also claimed that there were no significant differences between treatment groups in regard to discontinuations due to adverse events. But in fact, in this study Lilly had used an innovation—an introductory phase in which children were exposed to Prozac, with those who had an adverse effect discontinuing before the formal trials commenced. The authors concluded that fluoxetine at 20 mg daily appeared to be well tolerated and effective for acute treatment of MDD in child and adolescent outpatients.

Lilly's application to the FDA included the two Emslie trials and a trial with children diagnosed with OCD. The FDA reviewer was Andrew Mosholder, who reported that the key Emslie study "failed to show statistically significant effect of fluoxetine according to the protocol specified primary outcome measure." Nevertheless, he concluded that "the supplement is approvable, in my opinion."[67]

FDA granted Lilly the requested six-month patent extension. In so doing, FDA painted themselves and other regulators into a corner. Whatever about accepting there could be a side effect like suicide, for most people licensing Prozac meant it worked and this could not be undone without the FDA being exposed to a charge of incompetence or worse.

Against this background, another study, the Treatment of Adolescent Depression Study (TADS), assumed huge importance. This study was published in late 2004, but FDA were aware of its key findings long before that—or at least the way in which the findings were going to be presented.

TADS was a large NIMH-funded study, making it supposedly independent of company influence. The lead author on the first publication was John March, and it had a range of other high-profile authors including Graham Emslie. It compared Prozac and Cognitive Behavior Therapy (CBT), and the combination of Prozac and CBT, with a placebo. The results apparently showed Prozac worked with no hint it might cause a problem.[68]

In total there were 439 depressed youths with 112 assigned to placebo, 109 to fluoxetine only, 111 to CBT only and 107 to a combination of CBT and fluoxetine, making this the largest paediatric study. It was a 12-week trial with follow-up to week 36. At the end of the acute phase and during the follow-up, several placebo subjects were switched to fluoxetine or fluoxetine and CBT.

Seven major publications stemmed from this study over the following four years, none hinting at any problem. All articles came with authors who were then, and in some cases still are, leading figures in the field.[69] There was a limited pool of child psychopharmacologists at this time and so many of these authors also feature on company trials claiming SSRIs work well and are safe.

The seven TADS articles all commented on the suicidality issue. Readers of this book reading any of these articles would be left with the impression there was no difference between fluoxetine and a placebo on this score. But of 42 suicidal episodes in TADS, 34 happened on Prozac and 3 on placebo.[70] No matter which way you cut the data, Prozac was much riskier than placebo.

Leaving aside the question of why a difference of this magnitude would be hidden, how can it be hidden?

Several tricks were used. One involved continuing to classify those patients who switched to fluoxetine and only then became suicidal as being in the placebo group. This is a trick companies had been using since Pfizer and SmithKline's original Zoloft and Paxil adult submissions to the FDA in the early 1990s.

There is a school of statistical thought that supports the use of this approach. The idea is that for randomization to work properly, one must classify all outcomes under the heading of the original treatment to which a subject was allocated. This is called an intention to treat analysis (ITT), but even enthusiastic supporters of ITT would find what investigators did in TADS beyond belief. And where FDA officials had noticed this tactic in other studies, they flagged it as breaching regulations.

Why would a problem like this be hidden? The most likely explanation is that having approved Prozac, there was no way that FDA or Britain's MHRA were going to admit they were wrong and change its status. As Lady Macbeth said, "What's done cannot be undone."

Later when document after document had to officially recognize SSRIs caused problems for adolescents they all claimed Prozac was exempt. Officially, there were simply no efficacy or safety issues where Prozac was concerned. But the only difference between the Prozac and Paxil studies is that one set got through FDA before the music stopped and the other didn't.

At the September PDAC hearings, John March was asked by FDA to present the TADS data. This was before the first paper was published. He claimed the data fully supported Prozac. The implication was that all SSRIs really worked, it was just that we hadn't quite cracked how to run clinical trials in children yet.

Study 329 and the FDA

Study 329 disrupted this Prozac narrative. Based on the submissions in studies 329 and 377, on October 10, 2002, Russell Katz, Director of Neuropharmacological Drug Products at the FDA, sent an approvable letter to GSK for Paxil in children.[71] The letter did request additional information about Paxil, but this is standard procedure. Crucially FDA were willing to avoid any mention in the label that Paxil had not been shown to work.

On November 14, 2002, faced with the scale of public concerns about paroxetine following the *Panorama* broadcast, a committee linked to the MHRA said it was convening a panel of experts to review the questions of suicidality and withdrawal. In preparation for the first meeting of this expert committee, MHRA officials met with GSK. GSK made no mention of any issues about lack of efficacy or adverse reactions in its paediatric clinical trials.

A week later, on November 21, the new ad hoc expert group began meeting with MHRA representatives. The meetings focused mainly on the problem of withdrawal reactions, although suicidality was also discussed. Healy was invited to present. He asked to have a colleague, Andrew Herxheimer, accompany him as a third party. This was turned down. Going into MHRA meetings without any control over what was reported about the discussions risked letting the MHRA later maintain to the public that it had listened to Healy and countered his arguments, even if it hadn't. Acting on a tip-off, Healy phoned a company in London that specialized in supplying listening devices for secret operations. Thirty minutes after settling on a choice of listening device, June Raine of the MHRA called to say that Healy could bring Dr. Herxheimer with him to the meeting.

Many members of MHRAs expert group had clear and declared conflicts of interest. The group was disbanded soon afterwards, ostensibly because one of the experts had undeclared conflicts of interest. Despite this, the committee concluded that no change in the warnings about suicide were necessary.

At this point, GSK still planned to submit paroxetine for approval for use with young people in Britain. On October 25, 2002, it had indicated in a submission to MHRA that "there was no signal identified as regards suicidality revealed by these analyses." On February 28, the company sent additional data on paroxetine and suicidal behaviour to the regulator. It was only after this MHRA realized GSK's submission had merged adult and paediatric adverse event data and failed to identify or differentiate between them. This was sharp practice.

In the "Emails from the Edge" broadcast on May 11, 2003, GSK's Alastair Benbow, head of European Clinical Psychiatry, appeared to admit that the company knew its studies showed that more people are suicidal on Seroxat/Paxil than on a placebo, but nevertheless insisted that "the illness is the problem":

> BENBOW: *Whilst self-harm and suicidal thoughts are clearly a feature of depression, they have not been shown in carefully done studies to be a feature of treatment with these medicines.*
>
> JOFRE: *Well in the carefully done study, it was the biggest study of its kind in America, more children became suicidal on Seroxat than on placebo—sugar pills.*
>
> BENBOW: *Yes, that may be true in that particular study, but if you look at —*
>
> JOFRE: *Well that's pretty worrying, isn't it?*

> BENBOW: *No, that's part of the pieces of evidence that we have to gather together to decide together with the regulatory authorities and obviously they are the appropriate people to assess this. They will look at all the data that's been generated in children.*[72]

"Emails from the Edge" kicked up such a storm that on May 23, the MHRA reconvened its Expert Working Group. At this meeting, GSK handed out a briefing document, which showed an increased rate of events relating to suicidal behaviour among depressed children treated with Seroxat. Its defence claimed these findings were not statistically significant.

But for most people, an increase in events is an increase in events. On the basis of the new information provided by GSK, on June 10, the MHRA issued a *Dear Doctor* letter warning against prescribing Seroxat to children. At this time, it estimated that between 7,000 and 8,000 children and youths under 18 were being treated with the drug in the UK.

At the end of June, the Expert Working Group concluded,

> *The balance of risks and benefits for the treatment of depressive illness in under-18s is judged to be unfavourable for paroxetine (Seroxat), venlafaxine (Efexor), sertraline (Lustral), citalopram (Cipramil), escitalopram (Cipralex) and mirtazapine (Zispin). It is not possible to assess the balance of risks and benefits for fluvoxamine (Faverin) due to the absence of paediatric clinical trial data. Only fluoxetine (Prozac) has been shown in clinical trials to be effective in treating depressive illness in children and adolescents, although it is possible that, in common with the other SSRIs, it is associated with a small increased risk of self-harm and suicidal thoughts. Overall, the balance of risks and benefits for fluoxetine in the treatment of depressive illness in under-18s is judged to be favourable.*[73]

In September 2003, Wyeth issued a *Dear Doctor* letter stating that Efexor (venlafaxine) should not be given to children or teenagers as it has not been proven to be effective and had been linked with an excess of suicidal and hostile events.

Meanwhile, the FDA, which had issued an advisory at the end of June, by October had backed away from its position of concern. On October 28, the *New York Times* and *Washington Post* reported on the FDA's Tom Laughren as follows:

> *The FDA issued a public health advisory yesterday that makes clear that the agency has grown* increasingly skeptical *that there is any link between antidepressant use and the risk of suicide in teenagers and children.*
>
> *"I think probably that we have backed off a little bit from the advisory issued in June, which recommended against using Paxil," said Dr. Thomas Laughren, an F.D.A. official. "I believe* ***our position now is that we just don't know.*** *" [emphasis added]*

In December 2003, in preparation for the February PDAC hearing, the FDA posted the details of company paediatric trials undertaken on its website; the MHRA did the same. At this point few people, academics or others, knew how to consult a website, so this was lost on most of the people interested in these issues. Nevertheless, the material made it very clear that of 15 trials done in children, all but the Prozac studies and one Celexa study were negative—and there could be doubts about all of these.

Back in Washington, on January 21, an American College of Neuropsychopharmacology report was released declaring that SSRIs are effective and do not increase suicide risk in people under 19:

> *"The evidence linking SSRIs to suicide is weak," said J. John Mann, M.D., Co-Chair of the ACNP Task Force. "There are strong lines of evidence in youth—from clinical trials, epidemiology and autopsy studies—that led the ACNP Task Force to conclude that SSRIs do not cause suicide in youth with depression."*

> *"The most likely explanation for the episodes of attempted suicide while taking SSRIs is the underlying depression, not the SSRIs," said Graham Emslie, M.D., Co-Chair of the ACNP Task Force... "The potential benefits of SSRIs outweigh the risks."*

Of the ten members of the ACNP Task Force, nine were paid consultants to drug companies that sell SSRIs. A short while later, seven came on the radar of Iowa Senator Chuck Grassley for failing to disclose to their universities all the payments they receive from drug companies, in violation of conflict of interest policies. Three were authors on Study 329—Wagner, Emslie and Ryan.

On February 1, the day before the PDAC meeting, the *San Francisco Chronicle* broke a story that Andrew Mosholder, an epidemiologist with the FDA, had been told he could not testify at the planned hearings. Having reviewed all the published and unpublished data on SSRIs, as requested by Russell Katz, Mosholder had concluded that the risk of suicidal events and serious self-harm was about twice as high for young people taking these medications. In his earlier review of paroxetine that underpinned the October 10 approvable letter, he had also found that "the three randomized, controlled trials in MDD [major depressive disorder], listed above, all failed to show a separation of paroxetine treatment from placebo on their primary efficacy measures."

In this case he noted,

> *The most prominent adverse reactions not seen in corresponding adult trials appear to involve behavioral effects; these events were coded with terms such as hostility and emotional lability. As previously noted, the sponsor's method of coding these events was potentially confusing, and thus additional information will be helpful for the purpose of definitively assessing the potential behavioral toxicity of paroxetine treatment in pediatric patients.*[74]

But at the February 2 hearing, the focus was on efficacy. Most of those present expressed surprise that first the MHRA and now the FDA agreed there had been 15 studies in children almost all of which were negative. In 2004, journalists and academics were discovering they could go on the MHRA website and see its assessment for themselves. The close to universally negative result was probably the most striking finding of the day.

The committee heard from 51 witnesses who were given three-minute slots. Among the criticisms of methodology presented at the hearing was the following by Dr. Irving Kirsch and Dr. David Antonuccio:

> *The effect of SSRIs is statistically significant, but it is not clinically significant… [and] these results were drawn from studies with design flaws that typically favor the study drug. For example, they frequently exclude placebo responders before random assignment, rely on ratings by clinicians who have a vested interest in the outcome, and are likely to be unblinded by medication side effects. Furthermore… adding unpublished studies, most of which have negative results, will surely shrink the difference between antidepressants and placebo even further… Clinically meaningful benefits (of SSRI use) have not been adequately demonstrated in depressed children. Therefore, no extra risk is warranted.*

This was an early rehearsal of an argument Kirsch later made in *The Emperor's New Drugs*[75] and in a *60 Minutes* program for CBS.

The emergence in mid-meeting of the document from SmithKline's Central Medical Affairs Team, which also spoke to efficacy rather than to safety, highlighted this concern. This document, combined with prominent accounts of the gagging of Andy Mosholder on the issue of suicide, made it impossible for the FDA to carry the day. Mosholder was very visibly in the audience at the meeting along with David Graham, the best known FDA whistle-blower.

PDAC members raised the question of uncertainty regarding the implications of different classifications for adverse events, including events relating to suicidality. This may have been a planted question as the FDA had a proposal in place even before the meeting to hand over the data to a Columbia University group under Kelly Posner.

> *Because of concerns about whether the varied events identified by sponsors under the broad category of "possibly suicide-related" could all reasonably be considered to represent suicidality, the FDA asked Columbia University to assemble an international panel of paediatric suicidality experts to undertake a blinded review of the reported behaviors using a rigorous classification system.*

Perceptions of the February 2 meeting may have also been coloured by an event a few days later. On February 7 Traci Johnson, a 19-year-old college student taking part in a healthy volunteer trial for duloxetine, which Lilly was trying to rush to the market as Cymbalta to fill the void left by Prozac, was found hanging by a scarf from a shower rod in the testing facility. Her story and photogenicity became front-page news.

According to the journalist who probed the story for the British newspaper *The Independent*,

> *Investigators from the Food and Drug Administration rushed to Indianapolis to determine whether the experimental drug was related to her death. The probe was inconclusive.*
>
> *This left researchers in a quandary. Was the drug safe or not?... When researchers and the press started asking about duloxetine, the FDA didn't scour its database and go public. It kept quiet.*
>
> *The FDA gave a legal rationale for its silence. Some clinical trial data are considered "trade secrets,"... and thus are exempted from release under the Freedom of Information Act... The trade-secrets rule can leave researchers in the dark about the most worrisome data...*
>
> *The argument for secrecy is that failed efforts at drug development need protection lest entrepreneurs suffer a competitive disadvantage when other companies aren't forced to expend the same time and money*

exploring dead ends... The problem is that many drugs have multiple uses. Duloxetine... is marketed under the brand name Cymbalta to treat depression. Traci Johnson committed suicide while taking duloxetine during tests for selling the drug to treat stress urinary incontinence, under the brand name Yentreve...

The FDA approved Cymbalta to treat depression in August 2004. By the end of that year, Cymbalta sales topped $61.3 million. At some point—the date is undisclosed—Eli Lilly began testing Yentreve. In January 2005, as Cymbalta sales climbed to $106.8 million for the first quarter, Lilly announced that it was withdrawing its application for Yentreve. Then it cited the trade-secret rule in refusing to disclose why the drug did not win approval. Perhaps the rationale was harmless—the drug didn't work for incontinence. But duloxetine has been approved as a treatment for incontinence in Europe since August 2004.[76]

The September black box hearings

The second set of FDA hearings was scheduled for September 14. Five days before they began, Congress opened hearings on the gagging of Andrew Mosholder. Among other things, the congressional questioners explored Zoloft's paediatric OCD data and the suicide signal this had shown in 1996 (see Chapter 5). The FDA pleaded inability to find any correspondence with Pfizer on this point. There were lots of people who could have helped them out if asked.

A number of features of the reconvened PDAC hearings suggested FDA had originally intended to bury the question of warnings. Herschel Jick from Boston was called to present data that appeared to clear Paxil.[77] John March was called on to present data from the just about to be published Treatment of Adolescent Depression Study (TADS). This appeared to exonerate Prozac and by extension other SSRIs. The TADS study was still unpublished which made it difficult for anyone to contest March's message.

At the reconvened hearings, the committee concluded that there was a causal link between antidepressants and paediatric suicidality. The vote was 15 to 8 that a Black Box Warning label be placed on antidepressants for which data had been presented—Prozac, Zoloft, Remeron, Paxil, Effexor, Celexa, Wellbutrin, Luvox and Serzone.

A week later, Bob Temple, Director of the Office of Medical Policy at FDA, made a statement to the congressional committee, explaining why Mosholder had not been allowed to testify at the February 2 hearings:

> *While Centre for Drug Evaluation Research (CDER) was moving ahead with plans for the February 2, 2004, Advisory Committee meeting, Dr. Mosholder was nearing completion of his review of the data from the clinical trials provided in response to our July 22, 2003, request. Based on his review, he believed that the available data were sufficient to reach a conclusion about an association between the use of anti-depressants and suicidality in children and to recommend additional regulatory action, without the need for the more in-depth case classification or analyses that had already been initiated by DNDP [Division of Non-Prescription Drug Products].*
>
> *Dr. Mosholder had shared his conclusions with his supervisors and with the DNDP / ODE I [Office of Device Evaluation] review team involved in reviewing this issue. The review team and Dr. Mosholder's direct supervisors did not agree that the available data were sufficient to reach a conclusion and believed that definitive action should await the re-analysis by Center staff using the Columbia data. There was a discussion within the DNDP / ODE I review team, as well as higher CDER management including Drs. Katz, Laughren, and Temple, as to whether Dr. Mosholder's scientific and regulatory conclusions on the data should be presented in some form at the February meeting, given that they did not represent the Agency's (but rather an individual staff member's) determination; it was concluded that they should not be.*[78]

He concluded his testimony with this comment:

> *The results of pediatric depression studies to date raise very important problems. First, the poor effectiveness results, except for Prozac, make it very difficult for practitioners to know what to do to treat a very serious, life-threatening illness. While we believe that these drugs may be effective in children, studies have not shown this to be true.*

Despite being forced into a Black Box, FDA had not given up the battle.

On October 3, 2004, *Panorama*'s "Taken on Trust"[79] eviscerated Alasdair Breckenridge, the head of Britain's MHRA. The message from the program—not from Breckenridge—was that "in due course we may look at all of this and think this was one of the biggest medical scandals ever."

On October 14, in a statement to a U.K. House of Common Select Committee hearing, Healy noted,

> *In the case of fluoxetine [Prozac], an early series of clinical trials failed to establish efficacy for this drug in treating childhood nervous problems. This work led to a study that started in 1990, which involved extensive pre-screening of patients so that less than one-fifth of those screened entered the study, and those who did were put through a placebo washout phase in an effort to reduce the high rate of placebo responsiveness found in SSRI trials in children using these procedures. [The November 1997 Emslie article] claimed that Prozac could produce beneficial effects for children and adolescents. However, in fact on the primary end-point measure, Prozac was no better than placebo and on secondary measures benefits were apparent on physician-based ratings but not on patient or carer ratings. In addition, there was a 29% drop-out rate on Prozac and the rate of behavioural side effects was greater on Prozac than on placebo.*

On December 6, MHRA's final *Expert Working Group Report on The Safety Of SSRI Antidepressants* was published. The MHRA had gone further than FDA in semi-banning the use of antidepressants for children and adolescents in June 2003—except for Prozac. It wasn't illegal to prescribe any of these drugs but was clearly being frowned on—until the coast cleared.

This report introduced a new gambit into the game. It reported on Young Adults (18-24) claiming:

> *The clinical trial data for each product was reviewed in relation to a possible effect in young adults, and the GPRD [General Practice Research Database] study looked specifically at this age group. From these analyses, the Group concluded that there is no clear evidence of an increased risk of self-harm and suicidal thoughts in young adults of 18 years or over. However, given that individuals mature at different rates and that young adults are at a higher background risk of suicidal behaviour than older adults, as a precautionary measure young adults treated with SSRIs should be closely monitored.*

For adults it said:

> *There is no clear evidence that there is an increased risk of self-harm or suicidal thoughts when SSRIs are discontinued. Evidence of a relationship between suicidal behaviour and increasing/decreasing dose is not robust; however, patients should be monitored around the time of dose changes for any new symptoms or worsening of disease.*[80]

In these statements, there is a repeated trade-off between efficacy and safety. The problem FDA and MHRA faced was not that there was a risk, but they could not in the case of children say the benefits outweighed the risks—except for Prozac.

In 1991, in negotiations with Lilly over the suicide risk of Prozac in adults, based on the data they had then, FDA proposed a class wide warning of suicide risk. A class wide warning would have meant Lilly would not have lost any market advantage.[81] The company resisted this. A warning would put a chill on prescribing these "effective" drugs and more lives might be lost as a result. Efficacy is a regulator's friend in these circumstances.

Just as posting trial data on the Internet was new, so too in 2005 blogs were a new thing. On December 26, the world woke up to a new blog under the title "1boringoldman". It caught attention because no one could work out who its anonymous author might be. He appeared to have a detailed understanding of events related to drug safety and conflicts of interest.

War in the trenches

Straight after the February PDAC hearing, even before the September hearings, a series of articles by Robert Gibbons, an epidemiologist based in Chicago, and John Mann, the co-chair of the American College of Neuropsychopharmacology Task Force, began to appear, claiming that the effect of warnings of suicide risk in paediatric populations had led to a drop in antidepressant usage and an increased rate of suicides in children. The data presented were loose in the extreme. As one reader later commented about yet another in a series of Gibbons articles,

> *In "SSRI Prescribing Rates and Adolescent Suicide: Is the Black Box Hurting or Helping?" (*Psychiatric Times, *October 2007, page 33) Gibbons and associates primarily use data from their* American Journal of Psychiatry *article that appeared in September 2007, in a not very veiled attempt to influence doctors and the FDA to roll back the "black-box" warning on the prescription of SSRIs for adolescents. One week later,* The New York Times *reported that this effort to link an uptick in adolescent suicide rates with the influence of the black-box warnings on decreased prescribing rates of SSRIs was undermined by data that showed that during the 2004 period in question, prescribing rates of SSRIs to adolescents had not yet fallen (Berenson A, Carey B. Experts question study on youth suicide rates.* New York Times. *September 14, 2007;1.).*[82]

As the skirmishing increased, in 2005 FDA called for companies to submit their adult data for review. At the time GSK was in close contact with John Mann, one of its most public defenders, over just what data to submit. In an April 3, 2006, news release accompanying an article called "The Flawed Basis for the FDA Post-Marketing Safety Decisions: The Example of Anti-Depressants and Children" by Donald F Klein, Mann noted, "Given that untreated major depression is the main cause of suicide in children and adolescents, and that suicide is the third leading cause of death among 15-to-24 year-olds, there is an urgent need for effective antidepressant treatments."[83]

One of GSK's questions to Mann was about one of the cards in their hand. In the late 1980s, Stuart Montgomery in London had persuaded Lilly to run a trial of Prozac in patients with what he called recurrent brief depressive disorder and GSK later called intermittent brief depressive disorder (IBDD) and most people call borderline personality disorder. Prozac bombed. An article was quietly published years later which gave no data on suicidal acts but conceded placebo had been dramatically better than Prozac in terms of benefits.

Meanwhile Montgomery persuaded GSK to run a trial of Paxil in the same group of patients, probably in some of the same patients. There was the same poor outcome. The trial was aborted after some serious suicidal attempts. Nothing was ever published. There had been much higher suicidal event rate on Paxil than placebo.

So why in the mid-1990s did GSK go ahead with a similar trial in a similar group of people that also produced a huge suicidal event rate.[84]

What the company was up to perhaps became clear in April 2006, when in a press release they presented the following data for patients on paroxetine in Major Depressive Disorder (MDD) trials and IBDD trials.[85] The data for Paxil in this release for the two IBDD studies do not tally with the published and other data. But in fact we can make the IBDD data for Paxil much worse—we can add 16 suicidal events on Paxil—and still get an astonishing outcome. Combining two sets of patients where Paxil has been unhelpful can transform it into a drug that saves lives and the risk of suicide vanishes.

SUICIDAL EVENTS IN PAXIL DEPRESSION TRIALS

	Paroxetine	Placebo	Relative Risk
MDD Trials Acts/ Patients	11/2943	0/1671	Inf (1.3, inf)
IBDD Trials Acts/ Patients	32/147	35/151	0.9
Combined Acts/ Patients	43/3090	35/1822	0.7

This paradoxical outcome is predictable. Knowing what a drug can do makes it possible to design placebo-controlled RCTs that use a problem the drug causes to hide that same problem. In every case where a treatment and an illness can produce superficially similar outcomes, this can happen or be made to happen. It is particularly easy in illnesses from Parkinson's disease to back pain and depression where we have reason to believe that not everyone has the same condition.

So GSK's question to John Mann was can you come the heavy on FDA and insist they accept these data as part of our adult data submission. FDA did accept the data but it's not clear what use they put them to. FDA's call to companies had already been weird. They only wanted results from people actually on treatment. They didn't want the week or two before the trials began where companies had a track record of illegitimately creating placebo suicidal acts caused by withdrawal from prior treatments. They didn't want any data from the weeks just after treatment ended which are among the most dangerous phases. And just exactly what trick FDA pulled off with the data in subjects over the age of 65 remains a mystery.

In April 2006, GSK issued a *Dear Doctor* letter stating that there was a statistically significant increase in the risk of a suicidal act on Paxil in adults and modified the Paxil label accordingly.[86] FDA was not happy and asked them to undo this warning.

There were clearly complex calculations underway because a few weeks later, in May 2006, in response to an FDA requirement, GSK sent a "Dear Healthcare Professional" letter stating,

> *Current prescribing information for paroxetine—and for all other antidepressants—contains information in the WARNINGS section... stating that "patients with MDD, both adult and paediatric, may experience worsening of their depression and/or the emergence of suicidal ideation and behavior (suicidality), whether or not they are taking antidepressant medications... GSK has recently conducted a new meta-analysis... of suicidal behavior and ideation... Results of this analysis showed a higher frequency of suicidal behavior in young adults (prospectively defined as age 18–24) treated with paroxetine compared with a placebo.*[87]

This letter conveys the message that it is the depression that is the problem, but also opens up the question of young adults—a group that the MHRA had flagged at the end of 2004.

On December 13, 2006, FDA convened another Psychopharmacologic Drugs Advisory Committee (PDAC) hearing, chaired by Daniel Pine, to

> *discuss the results of an ongoing meta-analysis of data on suicidality emerging from antidepressant trials. Historically, this has been an issue that has been examined by many organizations including the FDA in great detail over the last five or so years. The specific purpose is to look at newly available data that focuses on results compiled by the FDA in trials among adults where all the previous meetings we have spent time talking about data in children.*[88]

GSK, and perhaps other companies, had at least one more manoeuvre to throw into the mix. They drew a distinction between "central" and "local" trials. Central trials were trials that the main GSK company owned and ran. Local trials were trials run with GSK drugs, that GSK had data from, but which might have been run by GSK France for instance or some entity that could be regarded as not part of GSK central. These data didn't get to FDA and typically contained more suicidal events than the "central" trials.

Even with all these efforts to limit the problems, the adult data FDA reviewed show an excess of suicides and suicidal events on active treatment compared to placebo. The relative risk of a suicidal event on antidepressants, especially SSRIs, in 25—to 65-year-olds is almost identical to the risk in under 25s. There would almost certainly have been very many more events if the withdrawal data had been included. The difference between the adult and the under-25 data is that the under-25 figures were statistically significant—and of course there is an apparent efficacy in the adult data as compared to the paediatric data.

The committee opted to extend the Black Box Warning to cover 18—25-year-olds. This had all the feel of a political manoeuvre rather than a data-based decision. On May 2, 2007, the FDA indicated that makers of all antidepressant medications should update the existing Black Box Warning on their product labels to include warnings about increased risks of suicidal thinking and behaviour (suicidality) in young adults aged 18 to 24 during initial treatment (generally the first one to two months).[89]

Out out damn spot

In June 2009, after a long series of articles claiming the Black Box Warnings were costing lives, Robert Gibbons got to chair an Institute of Medicine workshop that brought together experts from industry, academia, government and advocacy groups to discuss the issue of managing perceptions of suicidality on psychotropic drugs. The participants were asked to examine and discuss currently available data, data analysis and the future of potential partnerships in the area of clinical trials involving the nervous system.

The planning committee for the workshop included: Bill Potter (Merck), an NIMH-based Prozac defender in 1991 who then joined Lilly; Robert Gibbons, University of Illinois; Charles Beasley, Eli Lilly; David Brent, University of Pittsburgh and a critic of the Black Box Warnings; Yeates Conwell, U of Rochester, networked into Tom Laughren; Walter Koroshetz, National Institute of Neurological Disorders & Stroke; Thomas Laughren, FDA, an official closely tied to harm concealment efforts; Husseini Manji, Johnson & Johnson Pharmaceutical; David Michelson, Merck & Co.; Atul

Pande, GlaxoSmithKline, Inc.; Philip Wang, NIH, an expert witness for GSK and voter against the Black Box Warnings

This meeting was billed as a consensus conference. Consensus conferences are supposed to bring proponents of differing viewpoints together in an attempt to find common ground, but there were no differences between these participants.

The National Academy of Sciences, the National Science Foundation, the Alzheimer's Association, Astra-Zeneca, CeNeRx Biopharma, the Department of Health and Human Services, National Institutes of Health (including the National Institutes on Aging, Alcohol Abuse and Alcoholism, Drug Abuse, and Neurological Disorders & Stroke; National Eye Institute; the NIH Blueprint for Neuroscience Research; and NIMH), Eli Lilly, GE Healthcare, GSK, Johnson & Johnson, Merck Research Laboratories, the Society for Neuroscience, and Wyeth supported the project. It was clearly important to a lot of people.

At the meeting, Gibbons recommended examining item #3 of the weekly Hamilton Depression Rating Scale—the suicide item—and the degree of suicidal ideation and planning according to four levels of severity, in addition to overall Hamilton weekly ratings to determine treatment responsiveness and suicide attempts. He and Charles Beasley of Eli Lilly, he said, were conducting a reanalysis of Lilly's RCT data to determine whether this approach improves suicidal ideation as a predictor of suicidality.

This he suggested was better than the approach taken by FDA in 2004-2006, even though this was exactly the approach taken by Beasley and Lilly to the issue of Prozac and suicide in 1991 in their *BMJ* article, and by FDA at the 1991 hearings. This approach was panned in 1991, with even FDA dissing it in 2004 and 2006.

A report came out of the consensus conference, stating in part,

> *This report has been reviewed in draft form by individuals chosen for their diverse perspectives and technical expertise in accordance with procedures approved by the NRC's report review committee. The purpose*

> *of this independent review is to provide candid and critical comments that will assist the institution in making its published report as sound as possible and to ensure that the report meets institutional standards for objectivity, evidence and responsiveness to the study charge.*

There was yet another "consensus conference" in March 2009 that featured many of the same participants, notably Charles Beasley, along with Herb Meltzer and other academics in collaboration with FDA and industry on the topic of suicidality. This meeting also expressed doubt about the warnings of suicidality. Its deliberations were written up in the *Journal of Clinical Psychiatry*.

These groups all appeared to be desperately grappling with a need to find some way to stop people—patients or doctors—believing the evidence of their own eyes. When someone becomes suicidal on an antidepressant and it clears up when the drug is stopped and reappears when the drug is started again, this is conclusive evidence that the drug causes suicidality. But over 20 years, following the original Teicher article, companies and their affiliated experts had deployed rating scale data, arcane classification systems for suicidal events, miscoding of events, misuse of statistical significance, and lack of access to the clinical trial data as ways to obscure this fact.

This activity all looked like a concerted effort to roll back the Black Box Warning. The only reason to think it might not be a "conspiracy" was that it didn't make much sense that people would want to roll back the Black Box, which had had almost no effect on clinical practice or the sales of drugs. Raising problems with a group of drugs then going off-patent had opened up the possibility for companies to sell bipolar disorder and mood stabilizers. Diagnoses of juvenile bipolar disorder had begun appearing in 2003 and 2004 and were now booming on the back of claims that if children became suicidal on antidepressants this was because they were really bipolar. The Black Box was good for business.

Gibbons "new" research gave rise to papers he published in 2012—without Beasley's name on them—claiming that Lilly had given him unprecedented access to their clinical trial data for Prozac and that this access had shown the drug was free of problems. [90]He had discovered that the company had been excessively cautious. It took an independent investigator, like Dr Gibbons, looking at the actual data properly to realise there was no problem. Archives of Psychiatry published the paper to much fanfare.[91]

Blogging about the 2012 Gibbons papers, under the title Anatomy of a Deceit, the still mystery blogger, 1boringoldman, zeroed in on the flaws in this "research":

> *Robert Gibbons and senior author John Mann published an article in the Archives of General Psychiatry with a conclusion running against the current:... Dr. Gibbons... has had a long-held interest in obsession with this topic of suicidality in children on SSRI antidepressants and the FDA's black box warning issued in 2004...*
>
> *Dr. Gibbons, who was on the the FDA's advisory committee that voted in favor of the black box warning, said he was very concerned about the validity of the data that prompted the affirmative vote. "The adverse event reports for suicidal thoughts and behavior showed a fairly small signal in children, but the prospective measurements showed no effect of treatment whatsoever. As a statistician, I put more weight in prospective data than these retrospective reports," he said. "The vote was 15 to 8, so some of the members of the committee, myself included, were not persuaded by those reports and felt that the black box warning was not warranted"...*
>
> *Well, I knew that wasn't right in a way that was irrefutable—I had a case. I had put an adolescent on an SSRI who rapidly developed akathisia with confusion, aggressive thoughts, violent outbursts, the whole syndrome. His Mom stopped the medication, and he quickly cleared. There's no question about what happened. So I knew Dr. Gibbons et al. were wrong. I saw it. And I knew about Dr. Gibbons before the article was published...*

Here's what kept me at it besides a suspicion of bias based on his history. The article had no data or specific reference to the data... He said the data was from the complete data from the NIMH TADS study, all the Lilly Trials of Prozac and all the data from the adult Wyeth trials of Effexor and that the details would be in a companion article coming later. I knew that there were two Wyeth trials of Effexor in kids. Why weren't they there?... I wrote asking for the data sources and his reply was coming-in-the-next-article.

So every time I sat down at my computer, I checked to see if the second article had been published online yet. I was indeed obsessed. The topic is a big deal, his results widely touted, yet the study itself was hidden in the fog...

It showed up in early March, and it was a surprise to me. I was awaiting it to find out where the data came from, but it hadn't occurred to me what it would actually be about. It was also running against the current. They found that the SSRIs were efficacious in all age groups and their benefit transcended depression severity. Well, that was bold and counter to the findings of all the other meta-analyses. All of that using the same studies others used. No, wait, there was one in there that was new to most of us. The list of trials contained a stranger—Lilly Trial LYAQ? It hadn't been in any previous meta-analysis [in fact I couldn't even find it at all]...

A commenter located a reference to it and I finally found it on a Lilly Clinical Trial site, listed under Strattera, not Prozac, because it was primarily an ADHD Study with Prozac as an add-on.

With the four child studies and the two Gibbons et al. papers in front of me, I found plenty to worry about in the child data. Not only were the two Effexor studies missing—they mattered. They both show no efficacy and they were listed in other meta-analyses as showing a high suicidality rate. And study LYAQ was grossly inappropriate in that only some of the subjects were even depressed [it was an ADHD study][92].

If this effort had begun as an effort to roll back the Black Box, the real fruit of the exercise may well have been the Gibbons experiment. Why roll out a set of publications that repeated a discredited 20-year-old article? Perhaps to see what might happen if companies took an argument about data access that had slowly been building up a head of steam since GSK agreed to post study summaries on the company website and stood it on its head.

Partly triggered by GSK's deal with New York State in 2004, companies were facing a push for access to their clinical trial data. It would be extraordinarily useful to be able to say, "Hey look—when independent experts look at our data they find there were even fewer problems that we have reported to the wider world." The only problem with this is that Gibbons couldn't let anyone else see the data he supposedly had access to.

Several experts wrote into Archives of General Psychiatry critiquing the Gibbons paper, but the journal refused to publish letters. Why? For journals, there is the tempting prospect on the one hand of a series of apparently data-driven Gibbons-type papers that appear to tick all the research governance boxes and will bring the journal huge amounts of money in reprint fees. The opposing choice would involve an article based on access to the original data from, for instance, Study 329. Such an article would garner the journal nothing in reprint fees and would risk tying it up in legal knots and might even put it out of business. If you were the editor, what would you do?

Clay Center

A study appeared in June 2014 in the *BMJ* that appeared to support Gibbons. This study of teen suicide by Lu et al, researchers at Harvard, claimed to have found a "33% jump in suicide attempts" among US teens after the FDA placed a Black Box warning on antidepressants.[93] There was an avalanche of media coverage, none of which cast the faintest doubt on these alarmist conclusions.

Dozens of experts wrote into *BMJ* to point out the study's weaknesses. The journal at one point even removed the online responses. The article is a good candidate for the most egregious article *BMJ* ever published.[94] How it had slipped past the research editor Elizabeth Loder, also from Boston, was then a mystery.

The study was supported by the Clay Center for Young Healthy Minds, which was founded at Massachusetts General Hospital in 2013 and immediately waded into press coverage of teen depression and suicide. Gene Beresin and Steven Schlozman, two Mass General child psychiatrists, are its figureheads. Beresin went on ABC News to promote the "study". He and Schlozman wrote an Op Ed piece calling on FDA to repeal the Black Box warning, which Beresin called "the next closest thing to prohibition."

The Clay Center is a media and communications project dedicated to "educating" journalists, policymakers and the public. It is not a treatment or research institute. It has close links to the American Foundation for Suicide Prevention, NAMI, the Action Alliance for Suicide Prevention, and the Anxiety and Depression Association of America, whose leading lights have been Nemeroff, Mann and Gibbons and who receive significant funding from Pharma.

It owes its existence to Landon Clay, a venture capitalist and head of a Boston investment fund called East Hill. East Hill focuses on biotech ventures. Jeremy Knowles, twice Harvard's Dean, was on its Board until his death. Knowles was responsible for the Harvard Brain Science Institute which is heavily involved in psychiatric research at Mass General. He also served on the boards of Vertex Pharmaceuticals, Biogen, Celgene and the Howard Hughes Medical Institute (HHMI).

Another large donor is Elizabeth Hayden, who set up the Hayden Fund, in memory of her husband. This is administered by the Boston Foundation, a block of philanthropic capital with a finger in many political and economic pies in the Boston area. Hayden worked with Beresin on his idea for a media center. She may have been the person who recruited the Clay family to the cause.

The Center names WBUR, the Boston affiliate of National Public Radio, as an affiliate. It has strong ties to WGBH, Boston's PBS-TV channel. Despite the "Public" in their titles, NPR and PBS now get less than 10% of their money from the taxpayer. Half is from corporate and foundation sources, with the rest from individual-donor fundraising.

Both WBUR and WGBH, like *Sense about Science* in the UK, are regarded as prime sources for "responsible" mental health information by the media, even though WBUR is also part of the Sinclair News stable.

The clincher?

On May 18, 2017, Chris Cornell, lead singer for Soundgarden, committed suicide. The media reported his wife's hunch that the Ativan he was taking had caused his suicide. On May 25 WBUR in Boston interviewed Kelly Posner, who had headed up the Columbia Suicide Classification group the FDA had turned to between the two PDAC hearings in February and September 2004.

Posner dismissed the link between the drug and suicide. When quizzed about the fact that her group had reported the data that led to the Black Box Warning, she responded that both the FDA and she knew there was no link but they were stuck with trials that were not designed to look at the issue, and FDA, being very conservative and super-concerned about patient safety, had been ultra-cautious and issued a Black Box Warning that was, strictly speaking, unnecessary. Posner was looking forward to the day when all the new and better designed research coming through the system would lead to the Black Box being removed, because it had led to terrible unintended consequences—a drop in diagnoses of depression and a resulting increase in suicides.[95]

None of Kelly Posner's claims are supported by the data. This interview seems to reveal the original game-plan. It would have been interesting if the interviewer had questioned Posner about whether or not any of the studies showed that the drugs worked.

CHAPTER 8

Calls for Retraction

The Keller Study 329 paper triggered another drama that took a decade to come to a head but when it did it changed forever the debate about access to clinical trial data.[96]

Among the first to raise concerns about the Keller paper was Dr. Alex Weintrob from Cornell. In a letter to *JAACAP* published in April 2002, he stated,

> *In view of practitioners' concerns regarding safety and, even more so, parents' concerns about side effects and adverse effects of medications, I would like to have seen a more detailed description of the adverse effects found in the 11 patients receiving paroxetine who withdrew prematurely. In particular, I am interested in the five patients who withdrew because of "emotional lability (e.g., suicidal ideation/ gestures).*
>
> *As I previously reported in a Letter to the Editor... and as has been confirmed anecdotally by some psychopharmacologists, there have been instances of adolescents on selective serotonin reuptake inhibitors who have cut themselves. (Whether this is related to induction of a manic state is unclear.) This effect appears to have been causal. A more detailed description would thus be appreciated, particularly whether the "suicidal gestures" included self-mutilation.*[97]

Mitch Parsons from the University of Alberta expressed similar concerns:

> *I was concerned... by the report that 11 patients in the paroxetine group suffered serious adverse effects. This was in comparison with five in the imipramine group and two in the placebo group. This finding would*

> *appear to be statistically significant, though this was not specifically addressed in the study.*
>
> *I took particular note of the statement that "Of the 11 patients, only headache… was considered by the treating investigator to be related to paroxetine treatment." I would like to know on what basis the investigator dismissed the possibility that emotional lability, worsening depression, suicidal ideation or gestures, conduct problems, or behavioral disturbance could be due to the paroxetine.*
>
> *In the past decade I have treated hundreds of adolescent patients with SSRIs, and in my view all of these mentioned adverse effects have been temporally associated with the prescription of SSRIs…*
>
> *I certainly believe that paroxetine and the other SSRIs are useful medications, and as stated I am pleased to have a reasonably encouraging study that supports their use. I would value future studies, however, that look specifically at the issue of behavioral or cognitive side effects. Reports of these side effects have circulated since the advent of SSRIs and continue to be controversial. I also suggest that the reviewers of this article should have questioned more closely the dismissal of these symptoms as being unrelated to medication. This is particularly true in light of the fact that this study was funded by Glaxo-Smith-Kline, the makers of Paxil.*[98]

Keller, Ryan and Wagner responded:

> *The psychiatric symptoms were chronologically related to a variety of situational factors, such as arguments with boyfriend and parents, torment by peers, medication non-compliance, and/or untreated comorbid disorders." The only additional safety comment they made was about cardiovascular events on tricyclics: "In our opinion, the SSRIs, including paroxetine, represent safer therapeutic alternatives to the tricyclic antidepressants… We agree that further studies are needed to understand more completely the role of antidepressants, including the SSRIs, in the treatment of adolescents with major depression.*[99]

Keller simply did not address Dr. Weintrob's question about self-harm. He dismissed without any clear reason the possibility that suicidality and other aberrations could be attributable to paroxetine.

In November Drs. Correll and Pleak from New York wrote,

> *It remains unclear why Keller et al. defined one of the two primary outcome measures as a HAM-D score of ≤8, instead of the commonly used ≤7. Moreover, the most widely accepted criterion of a 50% reduction in baseline HAM-D score was not reported separately, but collapsed with the HAMD score of ≤8 (p = .11).*
>
> *While neither paroxetine nor imipramine differed significantly from placebo on either self rating scales (parent and patient) or non-symptom measures (functioning, health, and behaviour), this negative finding is not detailed in the Results section and the clinical relevance of rating score reductions is not discussed...*
>
> *Although serious adverse effects occurred with paroxetine (n = 11) more often than with imipramine (n = 5) and placebo (n = 2), only one case of severe headache was considered to be related to paroxetine. However, a potential selective serotonin reuptake inhibitor (SSRI)–induced mood disorder... is of concern in those 8 cases (4 requiring hospitalization) with "emotional lability" (n = 5), "conduct problems or hostility" (n = 2), and "euphoria/expansive mood" (n = 1), particularly if subjects did not have comorbid externalizing conditions before paroxetine treatment.*[100]

Keller with James McCafferty of GSK replied,

> *The criteria for therapeutic response were defined in the report as a final HAM-D score that was 8 or less or a reduction from baseline of 50% or more. Dual criteria were selected for this study because the scores at entry could range from a minimum of 12 (set by protocol) to a maximum of 53 (highest scores for the 17-item HAM-D). Limiting response to either a 50% reduction or a specified cut point would impede patients at the lower*

> *end of the ranges from meeting the criterion… The potential for SSRIs to induce mood disorders is not clear. In the present study, there was a history of behavior problems in several of the subjects that recurred during treatment.*[101]

Another letter from Raza Silveira was left without a response[102]. Then in December, Jon Jureidini and Anne Tonkin from the University of Adelaide wrote. They were told their letter would be published six months later. They twice asked to see Keller's response while waiting. No dice. They wrote again:

> *We write to request that you reconsider your decision not to give us access to Keller et al's reply to our letter prior to its publication in the middle of 2003. Our letter raises significant concerns and impact on the standing of the journal and profession that we believe cannot wait 6 months for our further attention.*
>
> *We would not wish to pursue these concerns if Keller et al have successfully refuted our criticisms. We think it is important and urgent to know whether we are correct in raising concerns about journal standards. We therefore request that you forward us a copy of Keller et al's response as soon as possible.*[103]

The editor Mina Dulcan replied six days later:

> *It is not the policy of the Journal to share responses to letters before publication. We do not have a backlog, and your letter and the Keller response will be published as soon as our production process allows. This is not a debate. We are under no obligation to publish whatever rejoinders you wish to make (or your original letter, either, which was quite rude and accusatory). Your approach to this process leads me to believe that whatever Dr. Keller says, you will disagree. Our readers will see both letters and make their own judgments. Frankly, your haste seems odd, since the article was originally published in July of 2001. I find your adversarial tone and urgency tedious.*

You have not been appointed as the guardian of the Journal, or of the profession of child and adolescent psychiatry. Many highly expert child and adolescent psychiatrists were participants in that study, and others that were similar, and others equally contributed to the review process. In addition, the prescription of SSRIs for youth, not only in this country but around the world, far predated any research data on their effects with youth, so this article could hardly be blamed or praised for that trend.

I noticed that you are members of Healthy Skepticism. Is this organization backed by anyone we should know about, for potential conflict of interest?" [104]

Jureidini and Tonkin's letter to *JAACAP* was published in May 2003 with a footnote saying they were members of an organization called Healthy Skepticism:

The article by Keller et al. (2001) is one of only two to date to show a positive response to SSRIs in child or adolescent depression. We believe that the Keller et al. study shows evidence of distorted and unbalanced reporting that seems to have evaded the scrutiny of your editorial process. The study authors designated two primary outcome measures: change from baseline in the Hamilton Rating Scale for Depression (HAM-D) and response (set as fall in HAM-D below 8 or by 50%). On neither of these measures did paroxetine differ significantly from placebo. Table 2 of the Keller article demonstrates that all three groups had similar changes in HAM-D total score and that the clinical significance of any differences between them would be questionable. Nowhere is this acknowledged. Instead:

- *The definition of response is changed…*
- *In reporting efficacy results, only "response" is indicated as a primary outcome measure, and it could be misunderstood that response was the primary outcome measure… Given that the research was paid for by GlaxoSmithKline, the makers of paroxetine, it is tempting to*

> *explain the mode of reporting as an attempt to show the drug in the most favorable light.*
>
> *Given the frequency with which it is cited,... this article may have contributed to the increased prescribing of SSRI medication to children and adolescents. We believe it is a matter of importance to public health that you acknowledge the failings of this article, so that its findings can be more realistically appraised in decision-making about the use of SSRIs in children.*[105]

A reply from Keller, Ryan, Strober, Weller, McCafferty, Hagino, Birmaher and Wagner was published alongside. It fudged the secondary efficacy measures as a technicality—"as scientists and clinicians we must adjudge whether or not the study overall found evidence of efficacy." The data, they claimed, "provides a strong signal for efficacy."[106] They closed with the following:

> *Drs. Jureidini and Tonkin argue that the reviewers failed to understand and appropriately critique the article (and by extension that the editor was not up to the task) and that the authors of the original article swerved from their moral and scientific duty under the influence of the pharmaceutical industry. By extension, of course, they covertly argue that the reader who agrees with them is intellectually and morally superior while a reader who does not agree with their position shares the cognitive and/or moral failing of the rest of us. We say that this article and body of scientific work is a matter for thoughtful and collegial discussion and say, in addition, that their emperor has no clothes.*

The making of the emperor's clothes

In February 1998 the six-month extension phase of 329 was completed. Work had already begun on the analysis and writeup of the eight-week acute phase of the study. In October, a memo from SKB employee Jackie Westaway explained,

As you well know the results of the studies were disappointing in that we did not reach statistical significance on the primary end points and thus the data do not support a label claim for the treatment of adolescent depression. The possibility of obtaining a safety statement from this data was considered but rejected. The best which could have been achieved was a statement that although safety data was reassuring, efficacy had not been demonstrated. Consultation of the marketing teams via Regulatory confirmed that this would be unacceptable commercially...

SmithKline's Central Medical Affairs Team (CMAT) document, attached to the Westaway memo, was marked "FOR INTERNAL USE ONLY." This article included the following statements:

Target: *To effectively manage the dissemination of these data in order to minimize any potential negative commercial impact.*

Proposals: *Positive data from Study 329 will be published in abstract form at the ECNP (Paris, November 1998) and a full manuscript of the 329 data will be progressed.*

When this document came to light in 2004, it provided the basis for Skip Murgatroyd, Cindy Hall and Karen Barth Menzies of the Baum Hedlund law firm to probe GSK for further details. They were helped by Leemon McHenry, a surfing buddy of Skip's who was also a philosopher but who on hearing what was falling out of these lawsuits figured that the laboratory for investigating the construction of contemporary knowledge lay in legal offices like Baum-Hedlund. The depositions undertaken on Keller[107] and in particular the real author of Study 329, Sally Laden[108], revealed what had happened.

After SmithKline staff had written up a "Final Clinical Report" of the acute phase of Study 329, they contracted Scientific Therapeutic International (STI) to prepare the article for publication in a psychiatry journal.

STI advertised itself as:

> *a full-service medical publishing group specializing in the development of scientific literature and other resource media with direct application to clinical therapeutics" with a staff that "is intimately familiar with the drug development process and the best possible use of print material to create and sustain awareness for a given concept, drug, or group of drugs, using a fair, balanced approach that maximizes credibility.*[109]

Sally Laden, an associate editorial director of STI, took on the brief. She produced the drafts of the original article and coordinated the publication process, including responding to peer reviews and editor's comments, proofreading galleys and providing submission packages to Keller that included draft cover letters for journal editors. Despite claims that the "authors" determined the content of the article, it appeared that SmithKline and STI maintained careful control over the drafting and publication process.[110]

In December 1998, Laden submitted a first draft with its conclusion: "Paroxetine is a safe and effective treatment of depression in the adolescent patient. Further studies are warranted to determine the optimal dose and duration of therapy."

In a July 1999 memo sent after the first revision, Jim McCafferty, a SmithKline executive, made three suggestions for Laden. The two "minor" ones were (1) the article should not imply that most of the trial subjects have a family history and a diagnosis of major depression when they do not, and (2) the statement that there are unlikely to be any more tricyclic antidepressant trials because of expired patents, while true, is too direct and sounds too commercial.

The third, "major," issue he raised was that of safety. In the memo he wrote:

> *It seems incongruous that we state that paroxetine is safe and yet report so many SAEs [serious adverse events]. I know the investigators have not raised an issue, but I fear the Editors will. I am still not sure how to describe these events."*

In August 1999, the first copy of the article, complete with correspondence from Martin Keller was submitted to the *Journal of the American Medical Association* (*JAMA*) entitled "Efficacy of Paroxetine in the Treatment of Adolescent Major Depression, A Randomized Controlled Trial." *JAMA* was the preferred journal because it reached family doctors and paediatricians as well as psychiatrists.

Two months later, three peer reviewers flagged concerns about whether the study really showed that paroxetine was effective, and *JAMA* declined to publish. The peer reviewers "pointed to the low HAM-D cut-off, the [confounding] effect of supportive care, the high placebo response, the small or absent differences in rating scales, the significant incidence of Serious Side Effects with Paroxetine, and the inappropriately [escalating and high] dosing with imipramine."

Following this rejection, Laden wrote to McCafferty:

> *Dr. Keller submitted the manuscript to* JAMA *in early August, 1999. The journal elected not to publish the paper and notified Dr. Keller in November. In a conference call in November involving Drs. Keller, Ryan, and Strober and Jim McCafferty, the action plan itemized below was agreed upon:*
>
> 1. *Sally Laden and Jim McCafferty will summarize the reviewers' extensive comments and draft a memo outlining the changes to be made.*
> 2. *This memo will be circulated to all authors for their review and approval.*
> 3. *The current draft will be revised and circulated to all authors for review and approval.*
> 4. *The revised manuscript will be submitted to the* American Journal of Psychiatry.
>
> *Resubmitting this manuscript is our top priority, and we will be asking for rapid review when we send materials to the authors…*

At this point, the plan was to submit the revision to the *American Journal of Psychiatry*. In May the decision switched to the *Journal of the American Academy of Child and Adolescent Psychiatry* (*JAACAP*), a journal that claimed to have the highest impact factor in the field of child psychiatry. The reason for this change is not clear. At the time however, Graham Emslie, one of the Study 329 authors, was on the board of *JAACAP*.

Following the revisions, the article was submitted to *JAACAP*, whose editor was Mina Dulcan, a professor of psychiatry from Chicago. The revision did not address the safety concerns of the *JAMA* reviewers. Indeed, the version accepted for publication in February 2001 did not address the concerns of *JAACAP*'s own reviewers, which were:

- Whether or not the claim of persistent depression in the patients over the whole year was justified was never clarified
- The high rate of serious adverse events in the paroxetine group remained unaddressed
- The high drop-out (non-completion) was never properly explained
- Whether SSRIs are an acceptable first-line treatment was not considered, and
- The suitability of use of HAM-D for children vs. adults is not discussed

The article was published in July 2001 with Keller as the lead author along with 21 others, some of whom were among the biggest names in the field of psychopharmacology and child psychiatry.[111]

The only critical differences between Laden's first draft and the final published article involve changes in the way efficacy and safety results were reported. A SmithKline statistician objected that the claim that there were eight primary outcomes might mislead readers. This led to a substitution of the label "Depression Related" for "Primary." In the peer review process with *JAACAP*, the term "primary outcomes" was reintroduced. Even then, the primary outcomes were reported in a way that subtly and deceptively made one of the primary outcomes appear positive, allowing the claim for efficacy to be retained.

Similarly, the dramatic downplaying of serious adverse events (SAEs) in the first draft could not be sustained. McCafferty's concerns led to his preparing an additional paragraph to acknowledge these effects. But just prior to publication, his contribution was changed in a way that made paroxetine look less dangerous. This late change appears to have come from within SmithKline rather than from any of the named authors.

Prior to the study's publication in March 2001 GlaxoSmithKline was working with New York public relations company Cohn and Wolfe. In email correspondence to Cohn and Wolfe, GSK noted,

> *Originally we planned to do extensive media relations surrounding this study [329] until we viewed the results. Essentially the study did not really show Paxil was effective in treating adolescent depression, which is not something we want to publicize. However, we should prepare Q&A and key messages in case reporters do cover this study. The proofs would definitely come in handy.*

Despite this clear acknowledgement of lack of efficacy, the message crafted was that this was a cutting-edge, landmark study that demonstrated the safety and efficacy of Paxil in the treatment of childhood and adolescent depression.

In April 2001, an email from Sally Laden to GSK made the following request: "Marty Keller is a corresponding author and will need a supply of reprints. I anticipate that he will need a sizable quantity because of the importance of this paper. Probably in the vicinity of 500 reprints. Dr. Keller is wondering if GSK will fund the purchase of these reprints. ."

GSK paid for the reprints, which were delivered to Dr. Keller.

The month following the publication of Study 329, a memo was sent to all representatives selling Paxil, copied to Dr. Martin Keller. In it sales management for the product made the following statement about Study 329: "This cutting edge, landmark study is the first to compare efficacy of an SSRI and a

TCA with placebo in the treatment of major depression in adolescents. Paxil demonstrates REMARKABLE efficacy and safety in the treatment of adolescent depression."

Blood from a stone

In 2010 *BMJ* ran "Rules of Retraction," an article by one of its staffers, Melanie Newman, which covered the story of the many efforts to get Study 329 retracted, given what had come to light. Newman noted that retractions of studies are rare when compared to the number of articles published each year: "In 1990, five out of 690,000 journal articles produced were retracted, compared with 95 retractions out of 1.4 million papers published in 2008." It appeared that retraction was reserved for clear cases of scientific fraud and errors so serious that they undermine the entire premise of the research.

The story behind Newman's *BMJ* article opens up another view of what journals do and don't do. In late 2006, as *Panorama* was preparing to run "Secrets of the Drug Trials," about Study 329, Leemon McHenry and Jon Jureidini, in agreement with Fiona Godlee, the new editor of *BMJ*, were going to write the history of the Study to have it retracted.

As part of "Secrets of the Drug Trials," Shelley Jofre interviewed JACAAP Editor Mina Dulcan:

> JOFRE: *You don't think the actual study as it was published overstated the effectiveness and underplayed the side effects?*
>
> DULCAN: *Well, all of that is a matter of opinion to some extent. How much is over, and how much is under… I mean it certainly listed the side effects.*
>
> JOFRE: *It didn't list them very clearly, did it?*
>
> DULCAN: *It depends on what you mean by clearly…*
>
> JOFRE: *I have got the peer reviewers' comments on Study 329…*
>
> DULCAN: *From the journal?*

JOFRE: *It says the relatively high rate of serious adverse effects of the drug was not addressed in the discussion. Given the high placebo response rate, are these drugs an acceptable first-line therapy for depressed teenagers? The results do not clearly indicate efficacy for the drug. I mean, these are pretty damning comments, aren't they?*

DULCAN: *First of all, I don't know how you would have gotten that, and second, we often have several series of reviews, and on virtually any paper if you read the reviews that came in on the first version they might have very little to do with the actual published version, so I really can't comment on that.*

Don't you think they sound pretty damning?

DULCAN: *I am not going to comment on how they sound because they could easily be out of context...*

JOFRE: *Surely the whole point of randomized control trials is to try and work out quite clearly what the drug is doing and what the drug is not doing.*

DULCAN: *That is the concept, but it's not that simple.*

JOFRE: *Not trying to complicate things, but what is quite clear is that the kids on the drug were having more psychiatric side effects than the kids who weren't taking the drug.*

DULCAN: *That was reported.*

JOFRE: *It wasn't clearly reported and it wasn't accurately reported, and the conclusion was that this was a drug that was generally well tolerated. It looks like 10% of the children who took Seroxat self-harmed—started to feel suicidal...*

DULCAN: *I think unless you understand the clinical condition, sometimes as people are getting better they appear to be suffering more. That's how the phenomenon works...*

JOFRE: *Are you aware that 329 was ghostwritten?*

DULCAN: *I have no way of knowing that. It doesn't surprise me to know it happens…*

JOFRE: *Does it worry you? Do you think it matters?*

DULCAN: *Well, certainly, if I were an author I would not put my name on anything that I didn't feel was —*

JOFRE: *Well, now that you know that there were more serious psychiatric effects for the children who were taking Seroxat compared to placebo, it means that the study published wasn't accurate. Have you got any plans to publish a correction or even pull it?*

DULCAN: *We certainly have no plans to either pull it, you can't actually pull it. You could issue a retraction…*

JOFRE: *Why not issue a retraction, because it's not accurate? What is reported in that study is not accurate.*

DULCAN: *I think if we found something that was fraudulent, that data were invented for example, that would be something. This is a difference in interpretation.*[112]

McHenry and Jureidini's paper on Study 329, "Clinical Trials and Drug Promotion: Selective Reporting in Study 329" was produced for the BBC deadline. *BMJ*'s lawyers advised against publication. McHenry and Jureidini split the paper into two, one on selective reporting with the same title and another on industry-sponsored ghostwriting.

The selective reporting paper went back to *BMJ*, where it was reviewed by Elizabeth Wager, the chair of the Committee of Publication Ethics (COPE), but also a ghostwriter and a former Glaxo employee, and by Richard Smith, the journal's former editor.

Wager disliked references to ghostwriting, giving the impression that these things may have happened in the past. Smith suggested that *BMJ* would be sued. Both said there was nothing novel in the paper. Shelley Jofre wrote in to confirm she had seen evidence to support all the claims being made and that no one had threatened to sue the BBC after the program aired. *BMJ* again turned the paper down.

McHenry and Jureidini took the selective reporting paper to the *International Journal of Risk & Safety in Medicine*[113] and the ghostwriting paper to *Accountability in Research.*[114] They also wrote up their efforts to retract 329 and published this as "Conflicted Medical Journals and the Failure of Trust" in Accountability in Research (which hasn't gone out of business).

Soon afterwards, Mina Dulcan stepped down as Editor of *JAACAP* and Andrés Martin took over. AACAP members, especially Ed Levin, along with McHenry, continued to press *JAACAP* for retraction. Before stepping down, Dulcan said, "It is not the role of scientific journals to police authorship."

When Martin took over, his stated position was that he didn't create the problem; he inherited it from Dulcan. He declined to publish any letters about the study. AACAP declined a submission of the material scheduled for McHenry and Jureidini's first paper on the issues—the *BMJ* paper—for a conference presentation in 2008.

The Keller paper continued to be cited as positive evidence for using SSRIs. In 2008, Jureidini found 226 published articles that cited it and retrieved 207 of the 211 that were in English[115]. Of the 207 articles, 153 discussed efficacy with false claims about the efficacy of paroxetine in 68 of these 153 articles (44%), with the reader being at risk of concluding that Study 329 was positive in another 54 articles (35%). The 68 articles that perpetuated the false claims did so by one or more of the following approaches:

- Explicitly designating Study 329 as positive
- Claiming that Study 329 demonstrated the efficacy of paroxetine
- Falsely reporting statistical significance on a primary outcome in Study 329
- Including Study 329 in a group of positive trials indicating the efficacy of SSRIs.

Only 31 articles (20% of the 153 that commented on efficacy) accurately reported the efficacy outcomes of Study 329. Only 12 of these 31 were critical of Keller et al.'s reporting of Study 329.

Melanie Newman's article two years later in *BMJ* appeared to be an olive branch from Fiona Godlee. *BMJ* lawyers were happy for the material to be published if written up by *BMJ* personnel with GSK given an invitation to respond. In the article, Newman noted, "The International Committee of Medical Journal Editors (ICMJE) advises retraction in cases of scientific fraud or where an error is 'so serious as to vitiate the entire body of work,' implying that this approach should not be used in cases of debate as to whether data have been interpreted correctly."

In this case, it seems everyone was bending over backwards to assume good faith, and to err on the side of not retracting without overwhelming evidence of fraud. Study 329 was viewed as a case of undue optimism resulting in exaggeration rather than fraud—despite the fraud case filed by New York State. No one mentioned the children at risk.

Newman cited Wager as warning that cases should be judged on the transparency standards of the day:

"Things have changed in the last few years." The U.S. requirement, in place since 2008, for all trials to be registered, including their pre-specified outcome measures, will make cherry picking harder, she says. "For the editor who is trying to decide whether, in hindsight, acceptable highlighting of positive results tipped over into unacceptable misrepresentation, there is no authoritative guidance at hand."

Continuing the chase

At the beginning of 2011, Jureidini and McHenry published a further article titled "Conflicted Medical Journals and the Failure of Trust." They wrote,

> *Journals are failing in their obligation to ensure that research is fairly represented to their readers, and must act decisively to retract fraudulent publications. Recent case reports have exposed how marketing objectives*

> *usurped scientific testing and compromised the credibility of academic medicine. But scant attention has been given to the role that journals play in this process, especially when evidence of research fraud fails to elicit corrective measures. Our experience with* JAACAP *illustrates the nature of the problem. The now-infamous Study 329 of paroxetine in adolescent depression was negative for efficacy on all eight protocol-specified outcomes and positive for harm, but* JAACAP *published a report of this study that concluded that "paroxetine is generally well tolerated and effective for major depression in adolescents." The journal's editors not only failed to exercise critical judgment in accepting the article, but when shown evidence that the article misrepresented the science, refused either to convey this information to the medical community or to retract the article.*[116]

In April 2011, Jureidini and McHenry contacted each of the Keller authors directly, asking them to request that JACAAP retract the article in the interest of scientific integrity, noting that the conclusions have misled clinicians into believing that paroxetine is safe and effective for use in adolescents when clearly it is not. Michael Sweeney responded that he did care about the data being presented accurately and requested further information. Jureidini sent him copies of the papers on 329, but there were no further exchanges. No one else replied.

In May 2011, Stan Kutcher, now based in Halifax, was standing for Parliament. A local newspaper, *The Coast*, published a piece about his involvement in Study 329. His lawyers wrote demanding an apology and retraction. *The Coast*, an outfit with no resources, complied.

In October 2011, a group of 24 physicians, academics and journalists, including Jureidini and McHenry, wrote to the President of Brown University, Ruth Simmons, asking her to request a retraction of Study 329. The request was passed to Edward Wing, the Dean of Medicine, who responded:[117]

> *With regard to your request for memos associated with an internal review, any reviews the University chooses to conduct in response to substantive concerns are undertaken on a confidential basis. Memoranda, letters, messages, policy reviews, or other internal documents associated with a review are not available to the public. I would caution you not to confuse the University's policy of confidentiality with inactivity.*

Jureidini and McHenry wrote back:

> *We acknowledge that confidentiality of personal information is important. However, we think that you misunderstood our request. You have said that we requested "memos associated with an internal review", but we made no request for any such memos or any other confidential information. Rather, we asked for your help to address the fact that the Keller et al article published in the Journal of the American Academy of Child and Adolescent Psychiatry seriously misrepresented the efficacy and safety of Paxil for the treatment of adolescent depression and continues to be cited uncritically in the medical literature....*
>
> *We specifically requested—and we now repeat our request—that you write an open letter to the Editor of* JAACAP, *Dr Andres Martin, supporting our request for retraction of the journal article... it would be a clear indicator of Brown University's commitment to taking appropriate action.'*

The response from Wing was brief:

> *As I stated in my letter to you on November 14th, the University takes seriously any questions about the soundness of faculty-conducted research.*
>
> *The University will not submit a letter requesting retraction to the editor of the* JAACAP *for the journal article written by Dr Keller.*

In June 2012, GSK was fined $3 US billion by the Department of Justice. Keller retired from Brown. A September 2012 post by the staff writers at *Drug Watch* noted:

Study 329 has never been retracted, however, and its authors did not face sanctions. The universities they represented did not even issue a public acknowledgement of the danger their academics created when they published a fabricated study. Furthermore, the lead author of the study, Martin Keller, was allowed to quietly retire from his academic position at Brown University at the end of June and maintain the title of emeritus professor of psychiatry and human behavior.

Jureidini wrote to Andrés Martin at *JAACAP* about a retraction in light of the Department of Justice fine. In a blog post on December 21 entitled "Hide-and-Go-Seek," 1boringoldman outlined what happened:

It's always funny when small children try to play hide-and-go-seek by covering their eyes, but when grown-ups do it, it loses its charm. That's what Dr. Andrés Martin has done in his response to Dr. Jureidini's request that JAACAP *retract the 2001 Study 329 article. They had a perfect chance to do the right thing. They declined to take it:*

> *Thank you for your Letter to the Editor, submitted July 20, 2012, regarding Keller et al., 2001. Following the June 27, 2012 settlement between GlaxoSmithKline and the U.S. Department of Justice, the Journal's editorial team undertook a thorough evaluation of the article, the legal settlement, and related materials. The authors of the article were contacted and asked to respond to the questions and concerns raised by the settlement. After a comprehensive and extensive review, the Journal editors found no basis for retraction or other editorial action.*
>
> *Due to the nature of the concerns and serious consideration given to the situation, the evaluation process was quite lengthy, and we appreciate your patience while the editorial team conducted its review. The inquiry is considered complete, and as such, your letter will not be published in the Journal.*

He continued: I had also contacted the American Academy of Child and Adolescent Psychiatry prior to their recent yearly meeting. Rather than write the Journal, I wrote the outgoing president, the incoming President, and contacted the Ethics Committee. All responded cordially and assured me convincingly that the matter was under review. So I think I was more hopeful than most about what they would do. My logic was that the American Academy of Child and Adolescent Psychiatry itself was responsible for its official journal, but as we now see, it remained in the hands of the journal.

"The authors of the article were contacted and asked to respond to the questions and concerns raised by the settlement." It goes without saying that contacting the authors seems an odd way to go about an investigation, particularly these authors. For example, there's a deposition of Martin Keller about this study available on the Internet. It's 125 pages long, but easy to summarize: "If you think I did something wrong, you're wrong because I've never done any wrong things, and I don't specifically remember anything I've ever done." That may sound facetious, but if you have the stomach to read it through, you'll agree with my assessment. It's maddening. Neal Ryan, the second author is heading up the Back to the Future Project which maps the road ahead for the AACAP. Karen Dineen Wagner, Boris Birmaher, and Graham Emslie continue to grind out articles about psychopharmacology in children and are prominent in AACAP affairs. I doubt that anyone on the author list was excited about the embarrassment of a retraction, but we already knew that. So did the Editor, Dr Andres Martin.

Meanwhile, several of the members of AACAP brought the issue up at the annual meeting on October 22, 2014. The minutes: noted that Dr. Martin "reviewed the timeline of the lengthy process used to vet the allegations raised numerous times over many years and to decide whether or not to retract the article, which included consultation with the authors, experts in publications and publication ethics (the Committee on Publication Ethics

(COPE)), experts in the field (psychology, child and adolescent psychiatry, clinical trialologists, etc), a whole range of attorneys, and more. By July 2010, Dr. Martin finished his independent assessment. He felt the process had been done correctly. Letters to the editor to retract the article had no supporting information and the letters were rejected."

No specific findings from Martin's investigation were recorded in the minutes.

Ivan Oransky, cofounder of the Retraction Watch blog, put it trenchantly:

> *GSK agreed to pay a $3bn fine and you're [Martin] saying you had completely different results? Great. Show me." Oransky described Martin's silence as part of the "typical scientific playbook." "It has certainly been our experience that journals and researchers and institutions can be incredibly stubborn about failing to retract a paper, about ignoring calls, or not responding favourably to calls to retract.*

When the restored Study 329 was finally published in September 2015, the original paper, the basis of a fraud action and a $3 billion fine, remained unretracted. Study 329 became the first randomized clinical trial to have two diametrically opposed interpretations in print at the same time.

CHAPTER 9

Cisparent or Transparent?

As the quest to get Study 329 retracted gained momentum, another struggle took shape—an effort to access clinical trial data. In principle this should never have been an issue—if there is no access to a study's data, it's not science and no one should pay any heed to it.

Access to data began to become an issue in the 1980s when pharmaceutical companies outsourced the running of their clinical trials to clinical research organizations (CROs). The trials became increasingly large with multiple centres and later several different countries. This was not because the drugs or trials were better but because they were weaker. The more effective a drug, the fewer the subjects needed in a trial. With this move, the clinical investigators running the trials lost access to the data. It was more convenient to store in it a central location, rather than the office of the lead investigator (Marty Keller for instance). CROs took on the task of coordinating this. Few people know the actual location of any physical data. Wherever it is, Study 329 revealed that the authors of the Keller paper had never seen even copies of the data.

The *Panorama* programs brought Jofre and Bell into contact with the lawyers who had been fighting SSRI suicide cases, including Andy Vickery, the trial lawyer in the *Forsyth* case and later the *Tobin* case,[118] and the firm Baum Hedlund.

Baum Hedlund had started in Santa Monica in 1986 fighting aviation cases. The original partners were John Coale, Mickey Kananack and Skip Murgatroyd. Murgatroyd had been driving cabs around LA until spotting an ad one day for law school gave up driving and took up law.[119] They were joined by Michael Baum and today the firm is known as Baum Hedlund. The firm took on early Prozac suicide cases and along with other plaintiffs' lawyers found itself dangling in the wind when the *Fentress* lawyers cut a deal with Lilly. But the Forsyth family wanted to pursue an action and had the means to stay in the game when others dropped out.

Suicide on antidepressants was a sideshow for Baum Hedlund at this point. Bill Downey had handled the suicide brief, helped by Cindy Hall and Karen Barth Menzies. Skip Murgatroyd had retired after ten years in law, a wealthy man, but when Downey died of cancer just before the *Forsyth* case began, he stepped back in, and bitten by the bug made the SSRI cases his hobby.

The suicide cases looked as if they had disappeared after the verdict went against Vickery and Baum Hedlund in the *Forsyth* case. But Hall, Barth Menzies and Murgatroyd kept the flame alight. Hall crafted many of the reports during this period and filed the motions that kept the legal options open. Barth Menzies, hugely articulate, friendly and photogenic, became the go-to public face for their efforts. Over a six-year period, they built up a set of political connections that transformed the landscape of all legal actions against pharmaceutical companies.[120]

In the background, Murgatroyd began to root through the documents detailing company efforts to hide the problems. In a series of cases he successively deposed experts like Marty Keller and Neal Ryan, the then CEO of GSK John Paul Garnier, ghostwriters like Sally Laden and regulators like Bob Temple.[121] The problems of antidepressants and suicide provided the template for what we now know about the relationships between academia and industry, resulting in the *Sunshine Act* passed in 2010.

Three amigos

In September 1991, when Lilly took its clinical trial data to the FDA in defence of Prozac, the person who presented the data that apparently cleared Prozac was Charles Nemeroff, then a middle-ranking professor of psychiatry at Duke University. Nemeroff was beginning a climb through the ranks, at a time when industry support could transform a less-than-average academic into a key opinion leader. A decade later, he had become the Boss of Bosses and was head of the psychiatry department at Emory University, where—as it turned out—1boringoldman had been a faculty member.[122]

In 1992, Marty Keller, who had recently moved to Brown University in Providence, became lead investigator on Study 329. Keller at this point was another mid-ranking professor of psychiatry who made a name for himself as a key opinion leader for pharmaceutical companies, primarily because he claimed depression might need lifetime treatment.[123]

In 1991, Alan Schatzberg became the Chair of Psychiatry at Stanford University. At Stanford he helped establish a company called Corcept Therapeutics, whose great hope was that a drug called mifepristone (RU 486), used as an abortifacient, might be licensed for the treatment of psychotic depression. There is a biological rationale for this in that mifepristone blocks cortisol, which is elevated in melancholic and psychotic depression.[124]

Nemeroff was at Duke University in the 1980s when Barney Carroll was head of department. Carroll had made his name as the creator of the Dexamethasone Suppression Test (DST), a cortisol-based test that distinguished melancholia from neurotic depression. After Carroll retired from Duke, he moved to Carmel, close to Stanford. He was a natural contact person for Schatzberg about mifepristone. Another person who had just moved to California was Bob Rubin, who had been Carroll's closest collaborator in his cortisol research.

Healy and Nemeroff, as noted, were both asked to speak at a University of Toronto meeting on November 30, 2000, celebrating the 75th anniversary of the university's Department of Psychiatry. Healy had recently been hired by the university and was due to move there. Behind the scenes, Nemeroff had approached David Goldbloom, who had been on the interview panel that hired Healy, and intimated the university would do better getting rid of Healy. Company funds might dry up otherwise. The Department of Psychiatry was heavily funded by industry at that point.

The following morning, at a committee meeting of the American Foundation for Suicide Prevention in New York, Nemeroff told those present that Healy had lost his job. Healy was also in New York in a Pfizer archive looking at data showing healthy volunteers becoming suicidal and aggressive on Zoloft in 1982 and Pfizer acknowledgments its drug had caused this and that other SSRIs can do similar things. A few days later, Healy began to get a string of emails from Goldbloom, which ended with a retraction of his job offer on the basis that he would not be a good fit with the needs of the department.[125]

Healy's talk had glancingly mentioned he believed SSRIs could make people suicidal but acknowledged that most people didn't believe this. The problem in coming to a common view, he figured, lay in a general lack of access to trial data that he had seen as an expert witness in legal cases. In the absence of access to the data, the question of transparency and conflicting interests had become important.

Transparency and the *Sunshine Act*

Two years later, in November 2002, a Nemeroff article, "Treatment of Mood Disorders," was published in *Nature Neuroscience*.[126] It noted that "available antidepressant drugs are safe and effective" but claimed other approaches might lead to better treatment. It concluded that mifepristone, a transdermal lithium patch and milnacipran (an SNRI that the FDA had rejected) were promising treatments for mood disorders, without disclosing that Nemeroff had a significant financial interest in all three.

Barney Carroll and Bob Rubin complained to *Nature Neuroscience* about this conflict of interest. Getting no response, they approached The *New York Times*, and on August 3, 2003, an article entitled "Physicians Raise Concerns About Undisclosed Financial Ties Between Researcher and Pharmaceutical Companies" publicly noted Nemeroff's conflict of interest, "Rubin and Carroll said that they sent a letter to the editors of the *Nature* journals in February to ask them to publish a letter that outlined Nemeroff's conflicts of interest. They said that they have not received a response."[127]

A month later, the editors of the *Nature* group of publications announced a change in editorial policy requiring that all conflicts of interest be disclosed. They noted that Nemeroff had not violated the policy in place in 2002. But this was a back-handed acknowledgement that up till then reviews that look like scientific analysis might be biased product promotions with readers being unaware of this fact. A month later, *Nature Neuroscience* finally published an editorial on Carroll and Rubin's concerns.[128]

Nemeroff soon after became editor of the American College of Neuropsychopharmacology journal, *Neuropsychopharmacology*. In 2006, his journal published a review article on Vagus Nerve Stimulation (VNS) authored by him with seven co-authors. Six of the co-authors were members of the advisory committee to Cyberonics,[129] the company producing the Vagus Nerve Stimulator, and the seventh was an employee at Cyberonics. Thanks were noted at the end for editorial assistance from Sally Laden.

Carroll and Rubin alerted ACNP to this conflict of interest; ACNP ignored them. They took the material to *The Wall Street Journal*,[130] whose story was picked up by *The New York Times*.[131] It became an international cause célèbre. ACNP eventually acknowledged the conflict of interest,[132] and Nemeroff was asked to step down as editor of the journal.

Parallel to this, in 2002, Schatzberg published an article in *Biological Psychiatry* on the benefit of mifepristone in psychotic depression.[133] The data did not support the claims made in the paper that mifepristone was an effective treatment for psychotic depression. The paper also failed to note Schatzberg's links to Corcept Therapeutics, which hoped to market mifepristone.

Carroll and Rubin wrote to *Biological Psychiatry*, but their letter was not published. They presented a poster at an ACNP meeting showing the data and the undeclared conflicts of interest. This kicked off a year-long tussle with ACNP, which was picked up by the *San Jose Mercury* in 2006, and again made headline news.[134] These events made Nemeroff and Schatzberg the poster figures for conflict of interest within medicine.[135]

On August 10, 2007, in a lawsuit, *O'Neal vs SmithKline Beecham,* Dr. Joseph Glenmullen filed a report containing the evidence collected by Baum Hedlund over more than a decade of cases involving problems with Paxil, culminating in GSK's April 2006 press release about Paxil and suicidal acts in depression trials. The case centred on the suicide of 13-year-old Benjamin Bratt while taking Paxil. The judge dismissed it on the basis that if the FDA had approved a drug's label, the manufacturer was powerless to warn about risks the FDA had not agreed to.

This bizarre judgement stemmed from company efforts to create a pre-emption defense:

> *In the 1930's, Congress became increasingly concerned about unsafe drugs and fraudulent marketing of drugs, and thus enacted the Federal Food, Drug and Cosmetic Act of 1938 ("*FDCA*"). The Act required new drugs to go through a pre-market approval process before they could be distributed. As part of the pre-approval process, the manufacturer had to propose a label which would have to be approved by the Food and Drug Administration ("FDA"). Importantly, when Congress enacted the* FDCA, *it was well aware of ongoing state tort actions over drug products, yet purposely decided not to include a private right of action for damages in the* FDCA *on the grounds that it was "unnecessary," because a "common-law right of action exists."*
>
> *In light of this legislative history, drug manufacturers rarely invoked the pre-emption defense and, when they did invoke it, it was almost always unsuccessful. That began to change in 2001 when, seemingly overnight, courts began to be deluged with pre-emption motions in prescription drug cases. In their pre-emption motions, manufacturers would generally argue that, since the FDA approved their product's labeling, any subsequent modification (including the addition of enhanced warnings) by the manufacturer would render the drug misbranded and subject the manufacturer to potential prosecution or enforcement action. Manufacturers contended that it would be impossible for them to comply with both*

federal law and state law (i.e., potential jury verdicts). Manufacturers further contended that a jury verdict would result in over-warning and, as a consequence, would stand as an obstacle to the FDA's accomplishment of regulatory objectives. Curiously, in a number of these cases, the FDA joined in the battle, filing amicus briefs in support of drug manufacturers. In 2006, the FDA also began making statements and revising its regulations in an effort to buttress the pharmaceutical industry's pre-emption defense.[136]

On September 6, 2007, Senators Charles Grassley (R-Iowa), the ranking member of the Committee on Finance, and Herb Kohl (D-Wisconsin), chair of the Special Committee on Aging, had introduced in Congress the *Physician Payments Sunshine Act*—so named because it aims to "shine a much needed ray of sunlight on a situation that contributes to the exorbitant cost of health care," according to co-sponsor Senator Charles Schumer (D-New York). The bill would require manufacturers of pharmaceuticals and medical devices with annual revenues of more than $100 million to disclose gifts or payments to physicians in any form, whether cash, trips or other.

In the wake of the *O'Neal* case, Cindy Hall contacted Grassley. This led to the unsealing on January 18, 2008, of Dr. Glenmullen's report, which reviewed the evidence collected by Baum Hedlund on the safety of paroxetine from the 1989 original submission onward. The report noted that in the case of many suicides, GSK did not attribute these to Paxil and had omitted them from the data. After reclassifying and reanalyzing the data, the report concluded that "Paxil increases the risk of suicidality in adults. In addition, GlaxoSmithKline was aware of this risk, but hid it."

Emilia di Santo in Grassley's office wrote to GSK asking how it was that it knew of the dangers posed by paroxetine in 1989, while the first the public heard of these dangers was the company's May 2006 "Dear Healthcare Professional" letter.

On June 11, Grassley wrote to Health and Human Services Secretary Michael O. Leavitt. He requested the FDA look into whether safety information had been withheld in the United States:

> *I have recently received an expert report prepared for litigation by Dr. Joseph Glenmullen, a professor at Harvard University. Based on documents from GlaxoSmithKline (GSK) and the FDA, Dr. Glenmullen concluded that GSK officials knew back in 1989 that Paxil is associated with an increased risk for suicide. I have attached his report for your review and consideration. Furthermore, I have learned that Britain's Medicine's and Healthcare Regulatory Authority (MHRA) concluded a four year investigation of Paxil. That report found that GSK had been aware since 1998 that Paxil was associated with a higher risk of suicidal behavior in adolescents. However, the British government did not move forward with criminal prosecutions because the laws at the time were not clear enough as to whether GSK should have informed the regulatory agency.*
>
> *In response to the MHRA report, Britain's public health minister, Dawn Primarolo, told* The Guardian *newspaper, "Companies that conduct clinical trials should not compromise people's health by withholding information."* The Guardian *also reported that the British government plans to introduce new legislation later this year to make clear that drug companies should not withhold safety information. In light of this investigation by the MHRA, I would like you to take a look at the information that agency gathered and determine if the company has withheld safety information here as well. I also request a briefing for my staff on whether or not a review is being conducted by HHS or any of its departments/ agencies regarding whether or not GSK withheld information from the FDA.*

These letters were about cisparency—access to clinical trial data. But Grassley's office, and in particular investigative researcher Paul Thacker, had been focused on transparency—the issue of payments from pharmaceutical companies to prominent academics. Schatzberg, Nemeroff and Keller were key figures given that so much about their conflicts was already in the public domain.

Rather than chase cisparency, Grassley continued with the low hanging fruit of transparency. The investigation scooped up Melissa De Bello, Joseph Biederman, Tim Wilens, David Brent, Jeffrey Bridge, Daniel Casey, David Dunner, Graham Emslie, Daniel Geller, Robert Gibbons, Frederick Goodwin, Andrew Leon, John Mann, John March, John Rush, Neal Ryan, David Shaffer, and Karen Wagner.

On July 12, 2008, the *New York Times* reported:

> *Now the profession itself is under attack in Congress, accused of allowing this relationship to become too cozy. After a series of stinging investigations of individual doctors' arrangements with drug makers, Senator Charles E. Grassley, Republican of Iowa, is demanding that the American Psychiatric Association, the field's premier professional organization, give an accounting of its financing.*

On September 24, 2008, CBS news revealed that "Dr. Martin Keller had been targeted by Senator Grassley and that investigators from the U.S. Senate Finance Committee were scrutinizing Brown University over disclosure of conflicts of interest in clinical research, Provost David Kertzer confirmed Thursday." The report continued:

> *Though university spokespeople would not comment on the details of a letter of inquiry from ranking committee member Senator Charles Grassley, R-Iowa, a source familiar with the investigation has confirmed that the letter names Professor of Psychiatry and Human Behavior Martin Keller, the chairman of the psychiatry department at the Alpert Medical School.*
>
> *Keller has gained notoriety for authoring a controversial clinical study of the antidepressant drug paroxetine—marketed as Paxil in the United States—which concluded that the drug was safe and effective in*

adolescents. Keller and some of the study's co-authors have been accused by doctors, lawyers, and journalists of having the 2001 study ghostwritten, earning large sums of money from Paxil's maker, GlaxoSmithKline. In addition, some say the researchers manipulated and suppressed data—including those showing increased suicidal tendencies in children taking the drug.

Study 329, as it is referred to by GSK, went on to become one of the most-cited articles in medical literature supporting the use of antidepressants for adolescent depression. At the time, GSK jumped on the favourable results, seeking to promote the use of its product among children, a largely untapped market for antidepressants.

Keller would later acknowledge in a 2006 deposition that he had been accepting tens of thousands of dollars in consulting fees from GSK and Scientific Therapeutics Information—a company acting on GSK's behalf—during and after the years he was conducting crucial research on the efficacy and safety of Paxil in children.

Alison Bass, a former reporter for *The Boston Globe*, said Keller may have earned more than he acknowledged in tax returns. In a 1999 article for the Globe, Bass reported that Keller had earned a total of $1 million in consulting fees from various drug companies over the fiscal years 1997 and 1998, according to his tax returns from those years.

According to Bass, the tax returns show that Keller received $218,000 from Pfizer and $77,400 from Bristol-Myers Squibb and that during that same year he had praised Pfizer's Zoloft and published positive conclusions on BMS's Serzone. Missing from his tax returns, Bass told *The Herald*, was the money Keller acknowledged earning from GSK.

On October 3, 2008, the *LA Times* reported that Senator Grassley's investigations uncovered the following:

A prominent Emory University psychiatrist received at least $2.8 million in consulting fees from companies whose drugs he was evaluating and *failed to report a third of it, congressional investigators studying medical conflicts of interest said Friday. The allegations against Dr. Charles B. Nemeroff, the latest in a series of such charges, are the most striking to emerge from the probe, which seems likely to alter the cozy relationships between prominent academics and the drug industry.*

Nemeroff received the money from GlaxoSmithKline between 2000 and 2007 while he was the principal investigator on a $3.9 million National Institutes of Health study of five Glaxo drugs for treatment of depression, Sen. Charles E. Grassley (R-Iowa), who initiated the investigation, said in a letter to Emory published Friday in the Congressional Record. Nemeroff continued to receive large amounts of money for delivering talks to other physicians even after he signed university documents pledging to accept no more than $10,000 a year from any one company, the inquiry found.[137]

Under the Title "Busted," 1boringoldman blogged,

In the mid 1980's, I was on the full time faculty at Emory in the Department of Psychiatry in charge of the Residency Training Program under an aging Chairman—a man who had founded the Department in the late 1950's. I was and am a Psychiatrist and Psychoanalyst, so my own interest was in psychotherapy/analysis, but we had a well-rounded program—or so I thought. When a new Chairman came from Duke, I liked him, but it became quickly apparent that whatever he thought Psychiatry was, it wasn't what I thought. After a year of being a fish out of water, I resigned, staying for a year to give myself time to figure out where to go next. I had tenure, so I had that luxury. After I left, this new Chairman became Dean of the Medical School and hired his friend Dr. Charles B. Nemeroff as Chairman of Psychiatry. The National Institutes of Health have strict rules mandating that conflicts of interest among grantees be managed or eliminated, but the health institutes rely on universities for oversight. If a university fails, the agency has the

> *power to suspend the school's entire portfolio of grants, which for Emory amounted to $190 million in 2005. But this step is so draconian that the health institutes almost never take it.*
>
> *Dr. Nemeroff was the principal investigator for a five-year, $3.9 million grant financed by the National Institute of Mental Health for which GlaxoSmithKline provided drugs. Income from GlaxoSmithKline of $10,000 or more in any year of the grant—a threshold Dr. Nemeroff crossed in 2003, 2004, 2005, and 2006, records show—would have required Emory to inform the health institutes and manage the conflict or remove Dr. Nemeroff as the investigator. Repeatedly assured by Dr. Nemeroff that he had not crossed this income threshold, Emory did nothing.*

Nemeroff left Emory and became Chair of Psychiatry in Miami in 2011.

Meanwhile, Business Week reported that Senator Grassley, as part of a congressional inquiry, said that Schatzberg, while Chair of Psychiatry at Stanford's medical school, had underreported his investments in Corcept Therapeutics, a company he founded. Grassley stated that Schatzberg had reported only $100,000+ investments in Corcept, but Schatzberg's investments actually totalled over $6 million. Stanford University indicated in correspondence to Grassley that it was "fully aware of the extent of Dr. Schatzberg's stake in Corcept Therapeutics" and that Dr. Schatzberg had "consistently disclosed on his annual conflict-of-interest forms his ownership of equity in Corcept Therapeutics in excess of $100,000 (the highest dollar category on the form)." Schatzberg voluntarily and temporarily stepped down as principal investigator from a related grant, which was funded by the National Institutes of Health. He was later reinstated.

On March 23, 2010, Grassley and Kohl's Physician Payment *Sunshine Act* was enacted as part of the Patient Protection and Affordable Care Act, which mandated companies to begin collecting data on payments to clinicians by August 1, 2013, and to have all data on payments publicly available by the end of September 2014.

There were increasing perceptions that a lot was going wrong in healthcare. For most ethicists, journalists and others, it seemed obvious what was wrong—the opinion leaders were being paid. Transparency was key.

In 2008, Healy was invited to give a plenary lecture on bipolar disorder at the annual ACNP meeting. Knowing Nemeroff was at the meeting, he kept an eye out for him and headed for him when he spotted him talking with a colleague. Healy extended a hand. Nemeroff looked flustered and scuttled off.

Cisparency

As part of the resolution of New York State's fraud action against it in 2004. GSK agreed it would post details of its clinical trials on a company website. This commitment led to the first clinical study reports (CSRs) being made publicly available. These were for the trials of paroxetine in children. The CSR for the acute phase of Study 329 was 782 pages long.

In addition to this, GSK posted summary reports of trials in other therapeutic areas, including trials of their blood-sugar-lowering blockbuster, rosiglitazone (Avandia). In reviewing the Avandia summary reports, Steven Nissen from the Cleveland Clinic, found that Avandia had an increased rate of mortality compared to placebo. Avandia was withdrawn from the European market and restricted in the United States. These data added to the basis for a Department of Justice action against GSK.

New players emerged in the debate in 2009. Peter Doshi from Johns Hopkins and Tom Jefferson from Rome, working with colleagues on a review of Tamiflu, Roche's antiviral drug for influenza, became headline news, when the data they assembled suggested Tamiflu didn't work. Doshi, a social scientist, had like Jofre and Murgatroyd an ability to see to the heart of an issue and to engage constructively with all points of view. Jefferson, an ex-army doctor and a family physician by training, had like another figure who emerged at this time, Peter Gøtzsche, an ability to call a spade a spade.

Governments around the world had stockpiled billions of dollars' worth of Tamiflu told it saved lives by reducing transmission of the virus, kept people out of hospital, and got them back to work faster. Over several years Doshi and Jefferson had asked Roche for access to their data, with the company agreeing but never delivering. With every study they did find, the case of the inefficacy of Tamiflu became stronger. Finally *BMJ* chose the Tamiflu saga as a clear-cut case on which to campaign for access to data (cisparency).

Doshi meanwhile had noticed that while GSK had agreed with New York to make data from its clinical trials available and it had indeed posted CSRs, the CSRs mentioned appendices A to H and these were nowhere in sight. In response to a letter from New York's Attorney General, GSK agreed to post Appendices A to G but not H.

Meanwhile in 2007, Peter Gøtzsche, the Director of the Nordic Cochrane Centre, asked the European Medicines Agency (EMA) to provide access to study reports on the weight-loss drugs rimonabant and sibutramine—both since withdrawn because of suicide risks among other issues. The EMA refused, citing commercial confidentiality. Gøtzsche argued the EMA was in breach of EU treaties. He appealed to Nikiforous Diamandouros, the European Ombudsman, and also applied to the Danish Medicines Agency for the data. In August 2009, he obtained some of the data from the Danish regulator. Diamandouros then required the EMA to provide access to all the data, and in February 2011 the data finally came.

Gøtzsche reports having had a lightbulb moment at a meeting on ghost-writing in Poland in 2010 when he became aware that beyond the reports no one, not even regulators, had full access to the actual data. He picked this issue up with Diamandouros and with a Danish Member of the European Parliament (MEP) Margrete Auken. When asked to talk on a different topic to the European Parliament, he persuaded Auken to arrange for him to speak about "Why we need easy access to all data from all clinical trials and how to accomplish it." At the Parliament he met Peter Liese, a German MEP, and came in contact with Transatlantic Consumer Dialogue. Their efforts resulted in a European Directive in 2012 mandating access to clinical trial data. A meeting was held at the EMA on November 16, 2012, at which the agency made it clear it was not in the business of offering unfettered access to trial data. [138]

As the European Medicines Agency was stalling, GSK seemed to be doing just the opposite. In July 2012, GSK agreed to plead guilty to criminal charges and pay a fine for promoting its antidepressants for unapproved uses and failing to report safety data about Avandia. A significant part of the fine hinged on Study 329. On October 26, the U.S. Department of Justice agreed to a $3 billion fine, the largest settlement for damages claimed in a Department of Justice lawsuit at the time.

Far from being on the back foot, GSK took the initiative, just as it had in response to Eliot Spitzer's 2004 lawsuit. It announced plans to make its clinical trial data available to researchers in 2013. The plan was to establish an independent panel of experts who would review information requests submitted by researchers. The company said it would then make data that the panel agreed met a scientific need available on a secure website.

A few weeks later, in January 2013, the birth was announced of AllTrials, a coalition whose proud parents were Sense about Science, the Cochrane Collaboration, the Centre for Evidence-Based Medicine, Iain Chalmers and several leading journals including *BMJ* and *PLOS* (Public Library of Science), with the lot fronted by Ben Goldacre.

The AllTrials ask was for access to the protocols for all clinical trials. The impression given was that AllTrials was seeking access to clinical trial data. It wasn't. It was named AllTrials rather than AllData. They support proposals that might enable some investigators, approved by companies, to access certain data. Exactly what GSK were proposing.

GSK promptly signed on to AllTrials. All of a sudden, within a few months of a record fine in the United States, Andrew Witty, GSK's CEO, was featured on the March 9, 2013, cover of *BMJ*, hailed as the acceptable face of the pharmaceutical industry.

At the same time, another company called AbbVie launched a legal action against the EMA, to block access to clinical trial data. Through 2013, GSK and AbbVie looked like the good and bad guys of the pharmaceutical industry. But in fact, both companies and AllTrials proposed the same thing—a "responsible" method of accessing a limited range of company data. Both asserted corporate privacy rights; both argued that access had to be restricted to ensure that patient confidentiality was not compromised.

The RIAT Act

On June 13, 2013, Peter Doshi, Kay Dickersin, David Healy, Swaroop Vedula and Tom Jefferson published an article in *BMJ* titled "Restoring Invisible and Abandoned Trials: A Call for People to Publish the Findings."[139] The first part of the title, expressing the authors' basic concept, was abbreviated to "RIAT."

Science Daily reported,

> *Experts are today calling for all unpublished and misreported trials to be published or formally corrected within the next year to ensure doctors and patients rely on complete and accurate information to make decisions about treatments. The* BMJ *is backing their call as part of its "Open Data" campaign…*
>
> *Unpublished and misreported studies make it difficult to determine the true value of a treatment. Around half of all clinical trials for the medicines we use today have never been published—and a whole range of widely used drugs have been represented as safer and more effective than they are, putting patients at risk and wasting public money.*
>
> *The authors of the declaration… will contact manufacturers of trials, asking them to signal their intent within 30 days to publish previously unpublished trials and formally correct previously misreported trials (i.e., to restore abandoned trials).*
>
> *They propose that if anyone who declares an intention to publish or correct does not do so within one year, all publicly available data for such trials should be considered "public access data" that others are allowed to publish…*
>
> *New freedom of information policies mean the public and the authors have access to around 178,000 pages of previously confidential trial*

> *documents and clinical study reports for widely used drugs for depression, heart disease, epilepsy and influenza. Some trials remain unpublished years after completion, while others have been published but have been shown to contain inaccuracies.*[140]

Given the amount of data that were available, Study 329 was the prime candidate for restoration. Jon Jureidini had been briefed on what was happening, and on April 26 he wrote to GSK CEO Andrew Witty, asking GSK to retract or request retraction of Keller et al.'s Study 329 paper or to restore Study 329 along the lines suggested by the RIAT authors.

On May 3, John Kraus responded on behalf of GSK saying no to the request for retraction, no to the suggestion that the reported findings were fraudulent, and no to the idea of rewriting the study. He noted that the study's authors had not requested a retraction, and the journal had refused other requests to retract.

On RIAT publication day, 1boringoldman blogged about the new initiative:

> *A bold remedy… To everything there is a season, and a time to every purpose under the heaven… Ecclesiastes 3:1, Corinthians II 6:2 In the story of every tension, there's a time for reflection and understanding, and then there's a time for action… The time for just decrying the shameful abuse of clinical trials in psychiatry and the rest of medicine has passed… The Cochrane Collaboration, Peter Doshi, and Tom Jefferson have been playing hard chess with Roche around the billion dollar efficacy questions with Tamiflu. Healthy Skepticism and others have dogged the* JAACAP *over Paxil Study 329 for a decade. Dr. David Healy's Pharmageddon and Rxisk database have taken on trials as well as adverse effects in general. Now comes RIAT [Restoring Invisible and Abandoned Trials] backed by a broad collaboration proposing a plan to add some teeth to the demands for clinical trial reform, focusing on missing and jury-rigged studies. The plan was announced today…*

The RIAT team drawn up to work on Study 329 included Jon Jureidini, Melissa Raven and Catalin Tufanaru in Adelaide, Elia Abi-Jaoude in Toronto, and Joanna Le Noury and David Healy in North Wales where it's too wet to do anything except work on something like this. It also included Mickey Nardo, a retired child psychiatrist who had worked in the Emory Department of Psychiatry but now lived in the backwoods in the hills of Georgia, where he kept his hand in by seeing poorest-of-the-poor patients and blogging.

Nardo picked up the efficacy issue with the help of Abi-Jaoude, also a child psychiatrist. Le Noury, a psychology researcher, and Healy, a psychiatrist, worked on the harms data. Jureidini, a child psychiatrist, along with Raven and Tufanaru, both in public health and epidemiology, worked on auditing the process, interpreting the data and finessing the politics with GSK and later *BMJ*.

Work began in July 2013 on the data from the CSRs for Study 329 along with Appendices A to G but not Appendix H. Appendices A to G contain the protocol and summary tables of the data from 329. These come to 5,494 pages. Appendix H contains the case report forms (CRFs), which come closer to the actual data.

In a series of letters from September 4 to November 8, Jureidini requested access to GSK's CRFs, Appendix H. These show anonymized patient-level data. The company declined to make Appendix H available.

On October 9, in "The Wisdom of the Dixie Chicks," 1boringoldman blogged:

> *Having looked at GSK's proposed process for access myself, it gives GSK the choice of releasing the data based on the credentials of the applicant and GSK's opinion of the worthiness of their research proposal. I don't want access to their IPDs [individual patient data] to do further research. I want it to check and see if they're cheating again like they've done countless times before.*

On November 12 in a *BMJ* editorial, "Putting GlaxoSmithKline to the Test Over Paroxetine," Peter Doshi wrote:

> *Blockbuster antidepressant paroxetine is no stranger to headlines. The drug is now back centre stage as requests for clinical data from one of its trials are testing manufacturer GlaxoSmithKline's commitment to full transparency.*
>
> *GlaxoSmithKline is leading the pack in its efforts to liberate access to its clinical trial data. It was the first major pharmaceutical company to sign up to the international AllTrials petition calling for all trials to be registered with the full methods and the results reported... But one group's request for data is testing the limits of GSK's commitment to full transparency. Jon Jureidini, clinical professor of psychiatry at the University of Adelaide, is leading a team to reanalyse and republish the results of GSK's study 329.*

Finally, in November 2013, when the RIAT team applied to GSK once again for access to Appendix H, GSK surprisingly agreed. It may have been because the team asked for access for audit purposes, and GSK's experience of FDA audits was so benign that they thought little could go wrong. The request had to be framed in terms of a research proposal, which meant it then had to go through GSK's data access committee—even though it wasn't for research. The committee agreed to allow access.

In February, GSK provided two members of the RIAT team, Mickey Nardo and Joanna Le Noury, with access through a portal with a triple identification access system to a remote GSK desktop that they quickly came to call the periscope. They could not download or print off the data, and the system routinely blocked them at regular intervals. Beyond that, Appendix H had over 77,000 pages with up to four different versions of some patients' records. It was cumbersome, at times a nightmare, but the work itself was very simple. A bunch of 18-year-olds could do it quickly and easily if they were allowed print off the material and spread it across the floor and look for patterns.

Six months after access was granted and fourteen months after starting the process, on September 7, 2014, a Restored Study 329 was submitted to *BMJ*, which a year before had all but insisted it be sent to them. Its authors had great hopes for their neonate.

If the restoration were published, Study 329 would be the first clinical trial to have two completely divergent analyses in print at the same time—one the subject of a fraud action and a $3 billion fine, the other the only study in a major journal that comes complete with a dataset that others can analyze. What effect would this have?

CHAPTER 10

Path to Publication

The *BMJ*'s 'guidance for authors' page states that:

> *The* BMJ*'s mission is to lead the debate on health, and to engage, inform, and stimulate doctors, researchers and other health professionals in ways that will improve outcomes for patients. We aim to help doctors to make better decisions.*
>
> *To achieve these aims we publish original research articles, review and educational articles, news, letters, investigative journalism, and articles commenting on the clinical, scientific, social, political, and economic factors affecting health. We are delighted to consider articles for publication from doctors and others, and from anywhere in the world.*
>
> *We can publish only about 7% of the 7000–8000 articles we receive each year, but we aim to give quick and authoritative decisions. For all types of articles the average time from submission to first decision is two to three weeks and from acceptance to publication eight to 10 weeks. These times are usually shorter for original research articles…*

Round 1

The restoration of Study 329 began in July 2013, starting with the CSR data tables that had been published on GSK's website. The numbers were transcribed by hand to a database, a task that led one team member to leave. Eventually, in February 2014, GSK granted access to the individual patient-level data (Appendix H) via the GSK Secure Portal, the periscope, enabling the RIAT team to examine a selection (34%) of the case report forms (CRFs) generated during the study, as well as enabling a detailed examination of the efficacy data.

By September 2014, analysis of the acute phase was complete, and the team submitted the first version of the "Restoring Study 329" (R1) paper to the *BMJ*[141]. The journal sent the paper out for review.

Typically, two people are asked to review and comment on a research paper. However, there were six reviewers for the "Restoring Study 329" paper—Florian Naudet from Rennes; Peter Doshi, associate editor of *BMJ*; Hilde P. A. van der Aa, a clinical researcher from Amsterdam; Sarah Hetrick, Senior Research Fellow, Melbourne; Ernest Berry, a safety and security consultant; and David Henry, a professor at the University of Toronto.

BMJ also wrote to GSK asking it if it would wish to review; GSK declined. Jureidini had already sent a draft to GSK, indicating that it would be preferable if the contents were not dispersed. GSK replied that it would not be telling anyone about the paper.

A *BMJ* editorial committee met on October 30 to discuss the six reviews it had received. The editor responsible for the paper was Elizabeth Loder, MD, a Boston-based neurologist. On November 3, 2014, an email from Loder kicked off *BMJ*'s correspondence with RIAT:

> *We recognise the value of this paper but we have not yet reached a final decision on it. We believe the paper needs extensive revision and clarifications in response to a number of matters identified by the peer reviewers and editors. We hope very much that you will be willing and able to revise your paper as explained below in the report.*

There were 130 comments and questions from the reviewers and editors. Although this sounds like a lot, in fact there was little of great difficulty raised by the reviewers, except one reviewer who was either not sympathetic or for whom the coin had not dropped.

From the start, the problems came from *BMJ*'s editors. Loder's letter highlighted what she viewed as the RIAT team's biases and conflicts of interest, barely mentioned by the reviewers:

> *We agree with several of the reviewers that the problem of potential bias and conflict of interest needs more attention. We would like to hear your thoughts about these matters and we think some comment in the paper itself might be necessary.*
>
> *Did the techniques used by the authors guard adequately against bias that might be introduced by their expectations, shaped by their previous experience of this study and related advocacy efforts?... Have the authors taken adequate steps to manage their professional conflicts of interest?... A number of the decisions that they made required judgments and I am not satisfied that they have taken adequate measures to avoid bias in making these.*
>
> *I was interested to know whether the reader should just believe that the Keller 2001 paper was ghost written or whether there is some kind of proof of this? How did the authors find this out/know?*

One of the barriers to accurately reporting adverse events from clinical trials highlighted by the revised paper lay in the "grouping of adverse events." In the original Keller et al. paper, all psychiatric adverse events were grouped, along with "dizziness" and "headache," under the class "nervous system" (see Table 3 in Chapter 2). The RIAT team proposed leaving "headache" in the neurological class, moving dizziness to cardiovascular, and putting the behavioural events in a new psychiatric class.

This simple move brought the psychiatric adverse events on paroxetine and placebo into view (see Chapter 11). The paper stated, however, that there was scope for others to parse these data differently. Access the data gives everyone a chance to reauthor a paper. Loder wasn't buying this:

> *We are particularly troubled by the recoding of adverse events. We did not agree, for example, that it makes sense to move symptoms such as dizziness and headache out of the nervous system cluster. I am afraid this makes us worry about other decisions that were made in the process of recoding. We agree with reviewers that coding of adverse events needs to be redone by people who are independent of your group.*

This was a great example of what the authors were up against. Headache hadn't been moved. The dizziness reported was all happening on imipramine, which drops blood pressure into a person's boots even at low doses, so the move to cardiovascular made sense. But the key point is that the team wasn't saying only one grouping was infallible. Other comments from the first round of reviews included the following:

> *Please present a true ITT analysis (in other words, analyze all subjects in the groups to which they were randomised, regardless of whether they received the study drug or not). Our statistician suggests that you consider having several columns in your results table. The first would present an ITT analysis using LOCF, the second using imputation and correcting for strata (12 centres). The third column could show the per protocol or complete case analysis using LOCF and the fourth the per protocol or complete case analysis using imputation. This would allow readers to judge for themselves the effects, if any, of using more modern methods of analysis, while still showing the originally intended efficacy analysis.*
>
> *We were disappointed that you did not examine the CRFs for all subjects. This seems a serious problem. It is, we understand, a major undertaking to review all of these documents, but seems necessary to set the record straight. After all, the trial itself was a major effort on the part of the original investigators*
>
> *I think that the change of coding between Lack of Efficacy and Adverse Event is difficult and could be misleading. Many times, discontinuation occurs for both lack of efficacy and adverse events, since one can easily consider that adverse events like dry mouth can be more acceptable in the case of treatment efficacy. This point could be addressed in the discussion and I'm not sure that an a posteriori interpretation of the CRF can give a perfect information about the individual patient experience (even if it is better than aggregated data of course…). Moreover, I also think that a lack of efficacy can be considered for patients even if they are responder upon the HDRS [Hamilton Depression Rating Scale].*

> *Patients are not just a score on a scale. The authors' a posteriori proposal for recoding this can be thus erroneous.*
>
> *Dr Loder also commented: We agree with reviewers that coding of adverse events needs to be redone by people who are independent of your group.*

The RIAT team was given four weeks to respond to these bizarre and *ad hominem* comments.

On December 2, Jureidini wrote to Loder indicating that the team would happily send representatives to meet with *BMJ* to show how the data from the reanalysis were collected and analyzed to help the editorial board understand what was involved. This offer was repeated on several occasions but was never taken up

His response covered all points raised by the reviewers. When reading these excerpts, readers should bear in mind that authors are in the position of a child being bullied by a parent or teacher or other authority figure. To get what they want they need to be polite.

> *Thank you for the exhaustive editorial and peer review of our important paper. It is the better for it. We have completed our response to reviewers and revised the manuscript accordingly…*
>
> *There remain three points of potential disagreement: the use of "more modern techniques" to analyse efficacy outcomes; the desirability of completing the analysis of CRF's; and whether we took adequate steps to ensure independence in analysing adverse events.*
>
> ***"More modern techniques" to analyse efficacy outcomes****—When it comes to efficacy, the point behind trials and statistical testing is to thoroughly test a manufacturer's claims because the well-being of vulnerable people is at stake. Trials are designed to weed out bogus claims.*
>
> *The contract under which GSK provided us with access to data specified that we were to follow the SKB protocol. This seemed appropriate. For a trial to be considered misleading, it should be by the standards that*

the initial researchers worked under, not "by modern standards." And we wished to avoid real or perceived bias in the way that we analysed the data… Using the protocol methodology, we could find no hint of efficacy. It is not our place to adopt ever more sophisticated methods to find hints of efficacy… If more "modern" methods of data imputation could have in any way retrieved this study, one imagines GSK would have done so… We ended up deciding that the choice of analytic technique was a potential source of bias (our own bias), and that in the efficacy analysis, we should wherever possible stick to the methodology prescribed by the original SKB a priori protocol.

Completing the analysis of CRF's**—***… We think it better that you do not require us to complete an analysis of the CRFs. When this Rewrite began, we had no expectation that we would get access to the CRFs… GSK were initially resistant to making the CRFs available. We did negotiate access to Appendix H (77,000 pages of CRFs, compared to approximately 5,500 pages in appendices A–G combined). But… the conditions under which GSK granted access were so restrictive that GSK's expectation may have been that we would be doing something similar to what FDA do, no more than dip into the occasional record to confirm that, for instance, individual patients existed… As events have transpired, our RIAT article has come to be about more than restoring Study 329. Once GSK granted access to the CRFs, the article has something very important to say about data access. It is unclear whether such access will ever be repeated; there is no commitment on the part of GSK to do this again for other groups.*

Apparently "completing" the evaluation of AEs [adverse events] direct from the CRFs risks doing a number of things.

- *giving the impression that the dataset was complete when there were at least 1,000 pages missing…*

- *giving the impression that using GSK's periscope is a reasonable approach to data access. In fact, neither we nor our readers really do have access to the CRFs in a meaningful way...*
- *distracting from what may be a major contribution to scientific debate—that there is no such thing as complete analysis, and conclusions from a trial are provisional and subject to improvement by others having equal access to the data.*

Analysing adverse events*—We believe it is important that the adverse event profile of both paroxetine and ultra-high dose imipramine, never before or since subject to valid testing in children, is provisional. We want to invite others, including GSK, to engage with this study.*

- *As noted in our submitted paper, the original protocol for Study 329 makes no mention of how AEs from this trial would be coded... blind coding is irrelevant. The blinding that counts is whether the clinician was blind to the drug the child was on when s/he deemed that child to be having an AE and used the clinical descriptors that now appear on the records.*

After that blind act, GSK coded these events. They may not have coded them blind. We used a much better coding system and coded blind. We did so because we anticipated the lack of understanding of readers who were not familiar with coding—we did not do so because the paper was methodologically stronger as a result of coding blind...

Across all codings, we would expect disinterested coders to rate our efforts more highly than GSKs. We have certainly done better than GSK did originally in this study where there are some very clear breaches of good coding practice... But the key point is this. If GSK engage in such an exercise, they will demonstrate the benefits of data access. Once there is data access, there is nothing to be gained by investigators (in this case us) being biased. We have a huge incentive to be genuine.

> *If you publish this covering letter written in response to the reviews, GSK will be put in an interesting position. If they don't already realise it, every effort on their part to draw attention to mistakes we have made on the basis of publicly available data that others can view will draw attention to the benefits of data access and the role of companies in denying access.*
>
> *We urge you… to publish the reviews as they stand and to wait and see if GSK (who are after all in the best position to carry out all kinds of analyses) respond by adopting the analyses proposed by the reviewers, and if so, what the outcomes are and what the scientific community would make of anything GSK offered in this area.*
>
> *In conclusion, we offer you a heavily thought out attempt that may provide a basis for setting a first set of standards for future RIAT efforts. In the case of an already published article, RIAT is not intended to be a conduit for criticism and bickering, but rather a serious and thorough analysis of the results of a study in a manner that aims at opening up rather than closing down debate.*

Round 2

As this correspondence took shape, a new Syriza government in Greece faced up to the iron fist of Germany in the velvet glove of a European Union. Greece had a credible deterrent—meet us half way or Europe's bankers will take a bath. In legal, moral and simple business terms the Greek proposals offered everyone a better deal. But it was clear from the get-go that their negotiating position hinged on every member of Syriza hanging together.

The same was true for RIAT. The exchanges between the RIAT team and *BMJ* from here on began to map onto the friendliness the Greeks showed on nightly news bulletins in the face of German snarls. This is standard in academia, where journal editors, who hold the power of publication, might know little or nothing about the issues, or worse yet might think they know something. Authors can always go elsewhere, but the editors assume they will buckle because they want publication in a prestigious journal. The difference here was that *BMJ* wanted this article at least as much as we wanted them.

There was silence until the beginning of February 2015, five months from the first submission. Jureidini requested an update from Loder, who replying the same day said that four of the original reviewers had been approached to "re-review," and the hold-up was because of one of these reviewers (David Henry).

> *As soon as his review is back I will decide, with other senior editors, whether the paper needs additional work, more discussion at a full manuscript meeting or whether a decision can be made immediately...*
>
> *I am very sorry things have not been speedier but we want very much to get things right.*

On March 4, 2015, six months in, Loder emailed,

> *I believe we are getting close to a version we will all find acceptable. At this point we are offering provisional acceptance provided you satisfactorily address the remaining points raised by reviewers.*
>
> *On other matters some changes are necessary.*
>
> *Deadline: Because we are trying to facilitate timely publication of manuscripts submitted to* BMJ, *your revised manuscript should be submitted by one month from today's date. If it is not possible for you to submit your revision by this date, we may have to consider your paper as a new submission.*

Attached to this letter was a second round of comments which, far from looking like the parties were getting close to agreement, seemed to take things back to square one and give a message of "do what we said months ago or nothing moves forward":

> HENRY: *This study has demonstrated that when there is access to primary data, trial conclusions will ordinarily be provisional rather than authoritative. I think that's a big call and too difficult to introduce in the*

abstract. Something like "the re-analysis of trial 329 illustrates the value of making primary trial data available" would be ok.

HENRY: *The authors state "only for six events from the eleven serious adverse event narratives was it not possible to be blind. This was 0.005% of events." I think we need to know whether the un-blinded assessment of these 6 serious AEs has a possible effect on the results—what do the results look like if they are removed? For instance what does Table 12 (Discussion) look like?*

These and other comments betray either a profound misunderstanding of what the authors were trying to do or else a simple obstinacy that could be drawn out until the RIAT coalition broke down.

BMJ's insistence on a statistical analysis that was never envisaged by the protocol for the trial was again raised as a sticking point:

Along with a number of reviewers and our statistical advisor I continue to think the paper would be stronger if you performed imputation. Performing these analyses would also demonstrate that you are doing your best to be fair and make the best and highest use of the data. There are arguments on both sides.

Loder was ignoring the arguments against carrying out this particular analysis outlined by her own reviewer, Peter Doshi:

Unless there is a strong argument that the statistical methods in the original study protocol are not just outdated but simply WRONG, I would agree with the RIAT authors' position that the analyses should be conducted according to the original protocol.

Every input from *BMJ* led to intense RIAT activity, necessarily spanning three continents and most time zones. On March 17, Jureidini replied to Loder:

Thank you for your second round of reviews and your offer of provisional acceptance…

It has been fascinating seeing how the paper has been read by the reviewers. While our goal with the responses has always been to address in full the reviewers' points, there has been a lot of learning about the process of authorship on the way…

Prompted by your reviewers, we have reworked the title and abstract to better reflect our view that our paper is as much about authorship and the authority of published conclusions as it is about the specifics of Study 329.

There is an important point related to blinding on which there appears to have been some confusion, hopefully now clarified. Dr. Henry appears concerned that non-blind coding of Serious AEs might have affected the findings. As per our previous letter, we are of the view that the original allocation needs to be blind—not the coding. The SAEs were coded blind. There were 6 "extra" non-serious events described within the narratives that were left uncoded or were coded and never transcribed. It was not possible to be blind to these, because allocation status was written into the narratives…

At least one of the missing events was a failure to transcribe 'Withdrawal Syndrome'. GSK had coded 'Withdrawal Syndrome' and 'Migraine' for one patient but only copied over 'Migraine' to Appendix D. Something similar may have happened for the other events—but this is less clear.

For those who think blind coding is important, we have had two MedDRA trained coders review a set of redacted SAEs. Both coders pulled out the additional 6 events that GSK had either left uncoded or not transcribed. We can supply the redacted SAEs to BMJ…

We hope that our responses, covered in more detail in our "response to reviewers" document, will allow BMJ *to proceed towards publication.*

> *If accepted, it would be great to get an indication from you for likely publication date.*

The key point in the growing tussle centred on the coding of the adverse event data. In 100 years of previous medical publishing, journals had never paid heed to this when reviewing a clinical trial paper. But all of a sudden, it was now crystal clear, as the team had hoped, that coding is a key act of authorship and the Restoration had laid bare the subjective component that lies right at the heart of this supposedly objective process. *BMJ* couldn't cope with this. It desperately sought objectivity, which for a journal really means some defence in case of a lawsuit.

The Restoration was also making it clear that adverse events were what pharmaceutical companies were most keen to hide. GSK had used a coding dictionary (ADECS) that no else ever used and was not even familiar to the FDA. The RIAT team used MedDRA, the Medical Dictionary for Regulatory Activities, which everyone now used, including FDA,[142] but *BMJ* strangely considered this an illegitimate move.

The team of authors uploaded the revised manuscript (R3) on March 20, with detailed responses to the second round of reviewer comments. Wherever possible, the team agreed with the reviewers and made the suggested changes and revisions, marvelling at their wisdom. However, on the issue of using multiple imputation:

> *we have thought carefully and decided against using imputation, largely for reasons that we have already set out. We note that we have the support of two of four of this round's reviewers, and that AW is in favour of imputation, but acknowledges contrary arguments, and that D Henry is silent on the issue.*

BMJ acknowledged the submission which was "presently being given full consideration for publication in *BMJ*."

Round 3

In the immediate few days following this third submission, the team received a string of positive sounding emails, including correspondence from the *BMJ* Technical Editor for Research, Vivien Chen, who wrote to Jureidini to explain that completing a checklist would be necessary to "prepare the article" for the *BMJ* "post-acceptance process." The changes required resulted in the submission of a revised manuscript on March 26, 2015.

A week later, Healy was deposed by GSK lawyers in the *Dolin* case, a Chicago action taken by the widow of Stewart Dolin, who had committed suicide six days after going on paroxetine. This was a problematic case for GSK and the entire pharmaceutical industry because Dolin had been taking generic paroxetine at the time of his death, as Paxil was off-patent, but the judge had agreed that as branded companies write the labelling even of generic drugs, Wendy Dolin should be allowed to sue GSK. The implications for all branded companies were considerable. At the deposition, in the interests of full transparency, Healy handed over the provisionally accepted Study 329 Restoration.

Ten days later, on April 15, having heard nothing, Jureidini emailed Loder to ask about the delay. She made clear the following day that the latest revision would once again be discussed at the next full manuscript meeting scheduled to take place the following week (April 23). On the website, the manuscript was no longer listed as provisionally accepted.

Far from the paper's being near publication, *BMJ* had sent the latest author responses to the reviewers again. A further two weeks passed with no further communication.

On May 1, Jureidini emailed Loder asking, "Is there some particular part of our paper that accounts for the delay? Something we could help with?"

Loder replied three days later and apologized for the delay. She explained that dealing with the first "RIAT" paper was a learning experience. She explained that further changes were recommended and noted, "We hope very much that you will be willing to make the changes that we recommend." In this latest letter, *BMJ*'s manuscript committee's "Decision" had now changed from "provisional acceptance" to "put points." She also provided detailed instructions on how to submit another revision of the paper.

The changes requested related to the relevance of the adverse events data, again the issue of the statistical analysis of the efficacy data, and the general "tone" of the paper:

> *The second point you make is about reporting and coding of AE. I am afraid we continue to find this less convincing, particularly the recoding of some of the AEs, especially given that you may be perceived to have a bias due to involvement in litigation. The sort of analysis you do was not specified in the original study and goes beyond what would have been done at the time of the trial. In fact, you use a classification scheme that was not in use when the study was done. It was also unclear why you do not do any statistical tests on the AEs. This is the least convincing part of the paper and no one felt it was fair. This really detracts from the main point of the paper which was the reanalysis of the efficacy findings, showing that the original claim of superiority rested on post-hoc outcomes. We continue to feel very uneasy about this because of the fact that you did not examine all case report forms. This is beyond your control, but it does reduce our confidence in the findings and is a major limitation. One editor commented that the emphasis on AEs seems like "the tail wagging the dog."*
>
> *We believe that you need to either present the AEs as they were originally coded and make fewer claims about them, or else ask completely independent investigators to code the AEs, report inter-rater agreement, and so on. It would only make sense to recode AEs, however, if you were also going to apply new methods to the efficacy data.*
>
> *Although we have told you that we will not require you to present results using imputation, we continue to think that would be useful. One of our editors, who had not previously seen this paper, asks "What is the purpose of the RIAT initiative? Is it (a) a way to beat the original authors over the head for misrepresenting the data? Or (b) is it an*

> *opportunity to see if reanalysis teases out findings that might have been missed the first time round? This is pertinent when considering whether or not to use imputation, and whether or not to statistically analyse the adverse events. Clearly if (a) above, one should stick with the original protocol, but if (b), one should go beyond the protocol." You would be on firmer ground in reclassifying the AEs using a new approach if you were open to doing the same with the efficacy data.*
>
> *Finally, we remain concerned about the tone of the paper. It should be neutral. In several places you stray into editorial comments about the difficulties of doing the analysis and so forth. Those things detract from the presentation of the research itself.*

BMJ was asking the authors to go back to a coding dictionary no one could find, which would allow for the coding of suicidal events as emotional lability and have these classified as neurological rather than psychiatric.

Jureidini responded, noting that it was unusual given that the paper had been provisionally accepted on March 3 that two months later new revisions were being requested along with suggested revisions that the RIAT team believed had already been addressed. He also stated that the team was not prepared to submit yet another draft for a prolonged review process with a new set of reviewers:

> *It is no longer clear to us if you still wish to publish the paper. If you are going to reject the paper, we want to know that within a week.*

Regarding her comment that "you may be perceived to have a bias due to involvement in litigation," he pointed out,

> *Your references to litigation are unfortunate. Involvement in litigation does have a potential for bias, as we have acknowledged, but it does not disqualify us from analyzing data. Unlike most other publishing in* BMJ *or elsewhere, we are exposing our biases to scrutiny by making all data available. There will always be potential COI in RIAT. The team has assembled for a reason. In the future, in any RCTs the* BMJ *publishes,*

> *will you insist that the coding is not done by anyone biased by their association with the trial, as sponsoring company or CRO or expert academics drafted in as notional authors, or indeed the clinical investigators themselves? Our rater was blinded and trained. We doubt you will find better quality control over the process of adverse events analysis and reporting.*

Regarding her comment that the emphasis on adverse events was like "the tail wagging the dog," he responded,

> *Far from our emphasis on adverse events being like "the tail wagging the dog," we think it is ground-breaking work that needs to be in the foreground, along with the fact that the paper is also a study in authorship and the effects of authorship on access to data. We are therefore unwilling to weaken our analysis.*
>
> *Second, we disagree with your implication that efficacy is primary, with harms being an adjunct. Historically, regulatory bodies were tasked with ensuring safety. Efficacy was added much later. Approving an inert non-toxic drug is a far lesser sin than approving one that works but is toxic. Consequently we focused heavily on harms, which were minimized in the original paper. As mentioned above, RIAT is explicitly about correcting the scientific record, including correcting reporting biases.*

He directed her attention to the rationale on this point previously submitted to the reviewers regarding "claims made about adverse events":

> *Please identify any claims that we make that are not supported by the data, and we will be happy to review.*
>
> *In our opinion, the point of the exercise is that making the data available makes it possible for others to have the kinds of concerns you may have and to argue your point of view. We do not want to stifle debate.*
>
> *If we can reach common ground on the AEs then I am confident we can resolve the other issues.*

In reply to concerns about "the tone of the paper," Jureidini stated:

> *We think we have been extraordinarily neutral in the circumstance, but if you indicate each episode of non-neutral language, we are prepared to have a go at flattening the tone further—from pancake to Kansas. (Kansas is technically the flatter of the two).*

The RIAT team agreed to make several other changes, including looking at the efficacy analysis:

> *With regard to imputation, we continue to hold that it is inappropriate to publish these results. However, if you insist, we will carry our multiple imputation and report it (preferably in an appendix), adding a note that this departs from the RIAT methodology and has been done at the editor's request.*

The team reiterated several times in the reply that it was willing to interact and negotiate, but it really now deserved a timely conclusion to the publication process:

> *We still want to see our paper published in the* BMJ, *and we request that you work quickly with us to a point of agreement to accept or reject it. We are happy to interact with and negotiate with you in order to accommodate a final rejection or acceptance within a week of your receiving this letter. At that point, if you decided to accept, we will submit a revised version within a week.*

Loder responded, "Thanks for getting back to me so quickly. I'll discuss this with the editorial team and let you know our thoughts."

Round 4

On May 21, Loder wrote to Jureidini citing the need for a legal review:

> *Many thanks for your patience in what I know has been an exhausting and tedious process of review and revision… I've had a long discussion with Peter Doshi about how to move forward with this paper. It is our intention at this point to make a decision in-house (without additional*

> *outside peer review) if we can agree on a few points. We will send the final version of the paper for review by our legal team.*

She mentioned the imputation analysis that she had insisted on previously and asked that it be included in the main body of the paper rather than in an appendix. With regard to her main concern regarding the coding of adverse events, she commented as follows:

> *It would work well to present both the ADECS and MedDRA adverse event data in the body of the paper, and acknowledge in the discussion the different interpretations that result from using the two systems. Please also provide more details in the methods section of your paper about the process of determining and coding the adverse events from verbatim term to preferred terms from CSR Appendix D. Who blinded, who coded, who assisted, did anyone double check the coding, how was blinding to drug assignment achieved... ?*
>
> *Can you also provide references or other information that will convince us that [your] process of coding is reliable, unbiased and reproducible?... The example you give about coding the scratch and emotional lability as suicidal ideation made everyone who read it worry quite a bit about the level of subjectivity that might be involved here—and I hope you are not offended if I say we felt that left everyone open to criticism given that you have acted as expert witnesses in court cases that presumably focused on AEs and harms.*

She concluded by noting that she looked forward to a revised version of the paper "if these recommendations are acceptable to you."

Jureidini responded the same day, enclosing a revised efficacy analysis and multiple imputation, which the team had been working on. In reply to Loder's other comments, the letter stated,

> *Our adverse event reporting is integral to our analysis of Study 329... We are committed to publishing the MedDRA coding and our analysis of it roughly as it currently stands... We are unwilling to use the*

original AE coding that scores suicidality as "emotional lability" or to hire an external rating team for AE coding, and we lack the resources to invest thousands of hours to examine all of the CRFs.

We understand your concerns about perceived COI in relation to David Healy's potential expert witness status, but we remind you that this issue has been present and public throughout the process of proposing the RIAT initiative, our writing this paper, and our dealing with the BMJ. *Also, as you know, our MedDRA rater was unconflicted and blinded, and the adverse event source data will be available for anyone to examine.*

If these conditions are unacceptable, we request that you reject our paper now, so that we can move on with publishing it elsewhere.

Things were becoming tense within the RIAT Team. Within the group views ranged between Mickey Nardo, who was inclined to give Godlee and *BMJ* the benefit of the doubt and viewed Loder as out of her depth, and Healy who figured *BMJ* wanted out. Healy constructed a written analysis of the *BMJ* comments including the following:

> BMJ *ask that we specify what was done to make the coding reliable, unbiased and reproducible… There is not a single other article about a clinical trial in the published literature that specifies these steps.*
>
> BMJ *have a primary concern—shielding the journal from a legal action… Along with this concern, their repeated insistence on adhering to items of the protocol (while at the same time blithely introducing imputation which has no place in the protocol) demonstrate the real trap… Conceding on imputation [is] one of those Janus things—two faces—good to be seen to co-operate, bad to have given them the impression that if they push we will buckle. GSK [and others] believe that a rigid adherence to analysis per protocol is the answer to all of life's problems… This is exactly what Andrew Witty's and industry's proposals for Data Access hope for… Data Access on the wrong terms would leave us all in a worse*

> *bind than now... companies [will be able to] design protocols in such a manner that the evidence from the trial can never come to light as* BMJ *are demonstrating here.*
>
> *The solution... is to make the data available... because a commitment to the data and its possible meanings is primary even though this means that bias is revealed and may be dissected in the process.*

The fourth revision of the manuscript (R4) was submitted on June 10. *BMJ* sent an email, noting that it "has been successfully submitted online and is presently being given full consideration for publication in *BMJ*."

Round 5

On June 15, Loder wrote to Jureidini with a second "provisional acceptance"—pending, however, further revisions:

> *We would like to publish it in the* BMJ *as long you are willing and able to revise it as we suggest in the report below from the manuscript meeting: we are provisionally offering acceptance but will make the final decision when we see the revised version.*

She specified that the provisional acceptance was conditional upon *BMJ* receiving the revised version within one month.

Towards the end of June, Loder advised Jureidini that:

> *I am writing to let you know that your paper is under legal review. I am afraid this is likely to result in a delay before any final determination can be made with regard to publication in the* BMJ. *I am sorry about the delay but I am sure you can understand the importance of this part of our process.*

The team was exasperated by the latest developments and indications that *BMJ* was pushing forward with another idea—taking on a third party to "independently review" the team's data collection and methods of analysis. We hadn't agreed with this. On July 6, Jureidini wrote to Fiona Godlee, *BMJ*'s Editor in Chief, saying,

I understand that you have now become directly involved in editorial management of our paper, and given how drawn out and difficult the process has been, I am taking the liberty of writing directly to you with a copy to Dr. Elizabeth Loder.

Throughout the ten month review process, we have responded promptly to BMJ*'s requests and been at pains to explain our analysis and other actions. It has now been three weeks since the most recent provisional acceptance from Dr. Loder, and we understand that there are no substantive issues with the content of the paper and that* BMJ*'s concern about the perceived conflicts of interest of some of the authors has been resolved.*

We understand… that you now want to check some of our data transcription and analysis prior to publication… We suspect that this level of checking is unprecedented. It seems to us that each time we satisfy a requirement, a new one emerges, and we have lost confidence that this "last step" will be the end of the matter.

In fact, it is not clear what BMJ *hopes to achieve by further checking our work.*

The team made another request to *BMJ* to accept or reject the paper. Godlee replied the same day:

I understand that the paper is largely now in a state that would be acceptable to publish and am grateful for the work you have put in to respond to the requests for revision. We also understand that most of the issues that the paper raises are already in the public domain…

However, it is our view that publication of the paper still carries risks… These risks are more editorial than legal… We have narrowed them down to one aspect of the study: the categorisation of the adverse events, and more specifically the self-harm and suicidal ideation. It is on this categorisation that we want to have independent checks… Yes, this is more than we have done in relation to other research papers we have published…

> *We believe that this checking could be done quite quickly... We are already seeking someone suitable to undertake the checks. Importantly they must be independent of you as authors and of The* BMJ. *Provided you are willing to continue to work with us on this, we will contact GSK as soon as possible to ask them to make their data accessible to the person we identify...*
>
> *We remain committed to your paper and to the spirit of the RIAT enterprise.*

Jureidini wrote two further letters to Godlee

> *Thank you for replying so promptly to yesterday's letter. However your response did not address some of our major concerns. How do you intend to resolve the inevitable differences of judgment that will arise in the checking process? What will be the mechanism for adjudicating whether any difference is problematic? How will you ensure that the data you receive from GSK will be identical to the data we have seen?*
>
> *We cannot see a way through these problems. As a result we fear that there will be further unacceptable delay in the publication of our paper.*
>
> *If you do have a mechanism for addressing these concerns, we need from you a clear time line to implement that mechanism, not just reassurance that it 'could be done quite quickly'.*
>
> *Finally, how can we be assured that that if this issue is resolved,* BMJ *will not find another issue that delays a clear final decision about acceptance or rejection?*

He sent a further letter to Godlee on July 9th:

> *...in our opinion the recent proposal you outlined for moving forward with publication of Study 329 is not feasible. Therefore, although our voluntary Study 329 RIAT team suffering from "submission fatigue this letter is an attempt to help (We could help more if you made it clear what constraints you are under and what concerns you.)*

> *"In an effort to facilitate resolution, we have revised our new Appendix 3, and added an accompanying set of notes in relation to the coding decisions for suicidal and self-injurious behaviour. We believe these documents will allow someone in* BMJ *or an independent scrutineer... to make a judgment call on the validity of what we have done. If whoever it is makes a good case that we have made a mistake, we will be happy to make changes. If there are differences of opinion, we would be happy to include words to that effects in a revised version.*
>
> *..We hope to hear from you by Monday with an acceptance of the paper as it stands, a rejection, an agreement to pursue one of the options we have outlined, or a detailed alternative with a clear schedule.'*

On July 5th the Greek people went to the polls and in a referendum resoundingly rejected German demands on their government. Syriza had the perfect mandate to hold tough but Alexis Tsipras, their leader, buckled. Varoufakis the finance minister, key to facing down the Germans, resigned. German obduracy had crushed the Greek rebellion.

On July 8th Jureidini wrote to Godlee, not copied to Loder:

> *I note your earlier comment about* BMJ*'s risks being "more editorial than legal." Coincidentally when we were looking up Dr. Elizabeth Loder's profile in relation to her concerns about our handling of headache in our adverse events analysis, we became aware of a potential conflict of interest.* BMJ *staff have understandably been very careful about any perceived conflict of interest on the part of our team, given that some of us have previously criticized GSK's Study 329; we now have concerns about Dr. Loder's indirect but significant links with GSK.*
>
> *Her hospital (Brigham and Women's) received over $12 million in research funding from GSK in 2014, up from just over $100,000 in 2003 (https://openpaymentsdata.cms.gov/company/100000005449).*
>
> *Dr. Loder has made public statements favourable to GSK products, including: "For all of these reasons my mantra is that 'You haven't failed*

> *sumatriptan until you have failed to respond to a full dose of injectable sumatriptan given early in an attack!' There is also evidence that combining a triptan with an anti-inflammatory drug might improve the likelihood it will be effective." (http://live.washingtonpost.com/how-serious-are-migraines.html)..*
>
> *This article was published just before GSK's Treximet (combination triptan and anti-inflammatory) came on to the market.*
>
> *Dr. Loder's husband, John M. Loder, is a partner in Ropes & Gray, a law firm retained by GSK in the US Department of Justice's action against them, in which Study 329 was a central element (http://www.law360.com/articles/250821/how-they-won-it-steptoe-gets-rare-acquittal-for-gsk--atty).*
>
> *More recently, the law firm has supported GSK with its difficulties in China.*[143]
>
> *Although, as Dr. Loder's COI declaration at* BMJ *points out, John Loder's work is not in the healthcare field, as a partner in Ropes & Gray, he presumably profits directly from such work. We believe that Dr. Loder's interests have been incompletely declared and that it might have been appropriate for her to recuse herself from involvement in the assessment of our paper to avoid any perception that GSK's interests were being considered in* BMJ*'s deliberations. While the timing for bringing these concerns to your attention is not ideal, we wanted to inform you as soon as possible after we became aware of these potential conflicts.*

In the course of the review process, Loder had made such a big deal about how headaches were being handled that, suspecting something, Healy did some research and became aware of her background as a headache-ologist. He bought her books on migraine and headaches in order to understand what was happening. In the course of this exploration, Healy and Le Noury came across her conflict of interest statement on the *BMJ* site, and from there her links to Ropes & Gray, and from there the links between Ropes & Gray and GSK.

This had become a duel. The July 8 letter to *BMJ* went unacknowledged.

Round 6

On July 17, Healy wrote to 12 other journal editors outlining the situation with *BMJ*, indicating his belief that *BMJ* was unlikely to publish and the RIAT team had a stack of reviews that could be made available along with the article to any journal interested in picking up an article that would be as high-profile as any journal could possibly wish. The expectation was that writing to so many editors would mean that at least one would report back to *BMJ*.

On July 19, Loder contacted Jureidini, stating

> *I am writing to let you know that we have identified a person to independently evaluate some of the outcomes. I am hopeful we will be able to issue a final decision soon.*

This independent reviewer was Tarang Sharma, a PhD student from the Nordic Cochrane Centre in Copenhagen. On July 29, enclosing a review by Sharma, Loder sent a letter to Jureidini requesting a number of changes. Once again, she noted that the RIAT team had one month to make the revisions and resubmit the paper.

She also suggested, "If you agree with the points our reviewer picked up on, we would like you to explain her assistance in the methods section of the paper."

One of Sharma's supervisors was David Healy, who was the source of a great deal of what she knew about coding suicidal acts. The idea that *BMJ* might request changes to what RIAT had done on her say was weird.

The RIAT team had been working on the harms data, especially the suicidal events, and Jureidini responded the following day with the changes the team figured might be helpful. He made no mention of Sharma.

At this stage *BMJ* was writing to the authors, who were responding with thanks for their comments but in fact paying no heed. In their view, *BMJ* comments had offered nothing to the paper for six months, but every interchange offered a chance to revisit the paper and make further additions that seemed useful. A sixth version was uploaded (R6).

Regarding the inclusion of the *BMJ*-elected "independent" reviewer, Jureidini responded,

> *We do not think the checker's contribution was as great as some other reviewers, for example Dr. Doshi. We will be happy for all reviewers to be acknowledged, and we propose that you make an editorial note about the extraordinary number and involvement of reviewers in this paper.*

Round 7

Over the course of the following days further "minor" queries regarding version 6 of the manuscript came back from *BMJ*. Loder commented,

> *I have some remaining minor requests. I will be checking my queue over the weekend so if you can make these changes quickly we may be able to have an acceptance decision before next week begins.*

Queries included a request to amend a couple of the figures and also:

> *In the methods section can you please indicate who decided how to allocate adverse events into system organ classes (SOCs) when doing the MEDdra coding? It isn't obvious why anorgasmia, somnolence, drug withdrawal and insomnia have been allocated to the psychiatric SOC. Is this specified by MEDdra or is it a matter of judgment? If so, whose was it? It is also not clear what is meant by the terms "toothache dystonia" and "sore throat dystonia" which are in the nervous system SOC. These things are in table iv in the appendix.*
>
> *On page 142 of 149 you say your analyses support the idea of drug dependence and withdrawal effects. I don't see convincing evidence of that in the paper. In any case, that also goes beyond the objectives of the original study or this reanalysis and should be removed.*

Over the weekend the RIAT team responded to all queries, and added, "We are confident that any remaining concerns can be sorted out in the copy-editing phase. It would be wonderful to hear from you by Monday."

Five days after the submission of the sixth version (R6), Jon Jureidini submitted a further revised manuscript. The seventh version (R7) incorporated some minor amendments.

On August 3, 11 months after the first version of the manuscript was submitted, Loder wrote to Jureidini,

> *Manuscript ID BMJ.2014.022379.R6 entitled "Restoring Study 329: efficacy and harms of paroxetine and imipramine in treatment of major depression in adolescence*
>
> *Many thanks for your patience with this very long process! I am delighted to let you know that your paper has been accepted for publication in the* BMJ.

Initially a date for publication was set for the first week in September. However, following concerns that some members of the RIAT team would be uncontactable in the week or so previous to this in order to approve proofs, the date was changed to September 12. Soon after, this was put back further to September 19. On August 28, Loder emailed Jureidini to suggest that the publication date be moved to September 26 to avoid coinciding with important Jewish holidays; the RIAT team vetoed this. Just over a year after the original submission, at 11:30 p.m. GMT on September 16, "Restoring Study 329" was published online, followed by print publication in the issue of September 19, 2015.[144]

Round 8

On September 30, Jureidini wrote to Godlee,

> *We have not received a reply to the... letter we sent you on 8 July, about our concerns about potential conflict of interest on the part of Dr. Loder. We still think that the issues we raised are important, so we are seeking a response from you.*

Godlee replied:

> *Thank you for your message. My apologies for not replying to your earlier message. I'm not sure how I missed it.*
>
> *Let me discuss your concerns with Dr. Loder. I will get back to you as soon as I have had a chance to do so.*

Nearly five weeks passed without any further correspondence. On November 4, Jureidini wrote, "Have you had chance to evaluate our concerns?" On December 14, he wrote again: "Just tidying things up before Christmas, and wanting to check if I will hear back from [you] about this potential COI issue."

Godlee replied two days later:

> *So sorry not to have got back to you about this, I referred it to our ethics committee which meets three times a year, but the last meeting was cancelled. They meet tomorrow and I should be able to give you their conclusion shortly afterwards.*

Then on January 3, 2016, she wrote,

> *The ethics committee's agenda was rather full for its December 16 meeting… and I am afraid we didn't get to this item. However, I have asked our chair, Professor Marion McMurdo, to convene an additional meeting, which I hope will take place in the next few weeks, in order that we can get you a response to your concerns.*

Godlee followed this up with an email on January 11, which contained a letter from Dr. Loder in response to the original concerns. This letter, dated December 16, 2015, said,

> *You asked me to respond to Dr. Jureidini's accusations of conflicts of interest regarding connections to GSK. These were 1) that my hospital, Brigham and Women's, receives research money form GSK; 2) that my husband is a partner in the law firm Ropes & Gray, which has done work for GSK and thus he profits directly from this connection; and 3) that I have made public statements favorable to GSK products.*

> *With regard the first matter, I don't keep track of nor do I have any practical way of knowing about the hospital's many sources of research support. BWH is one of the largest academic medical centers in the US and receives millions of dollars of research support from a vast array of companies and government agencies.*
>
> *With regard to the second matter, Ropes & Gray is a huge international law firm with thousands of clients. The firm has approximately 1200 lawyers working in 11 different offices around the world and well over $1 billion in annual revenues. I didn't have any knowledge of their work for GSK. My husband does not work in their healthcare division. He is a securities lawyer... Ropes & Gray's work for GSK and the firm's relationship with GSK accordingly had no influence on the editorial process.*
>
> *With regard to the third matter, the examples provided by Dr. Jureidini are taken out of context. They do not illustrate that I have spoken favorably about GSK products. You will note that in the live Q&A with the* Washington Post, *from which he pulled a quote, I use the generic name sumatriptan, and am answering a question by a reader who used the brand name.*

Godlee wrote,

> *The ethics committee convened on Friday 8 January. It was chaired by the committee chair Professor Marion McMurdo, attended by committee members Julian Sheather, Elizabeth Wager, and Dr. Adrian Sutton. Committee members who were unable to attend—Dr. Rubin Minhas, John Coggon, and Dr. Richard Hain—sent their comments by email. Also attending were myself, the* BMJ*'s Executive Editor Dr. Theo Bloom.*
>
> *The committee reviewed the issues you raised and, by a large majority, concluded that the possible conflicts you have identified are so attenuated by distance from Dr. Loder—by virtue of the size and scope of her and her husband's organisations, as to be highly unlikely to have impacted on her decision making. The committee felt that to require an*

> *individual to consider, manage, or declare such attenuated links would take declaration of conflicts of interest to an absurd level, since such potential conflicts would be near impossible for an individual to keep track of or to be held responsible for. The committee is satisfied with Dr. Loder's response.*

BMJ has a policy of uploading the letters from its editors, such as Dr. Loder, along with the reviews of an article and the responses of the authors, to sit beside the published article. To this day it has not posted the reviews for "Restoring Study 329." The letters, reviews and responses are available on *study329.org*.

Unlike Syriza, the RIAT coalition had held together but the strains had begun to show by July. The Syriza and RIAT dynamics were exactly the same. Those who wanted to compromise with the Germans figured that once a compromise was agreed the Germans would be reasonable. But diluting power with reasonableness is a recipe for loss of power.

What did *BMJ* really want? Whatever it was, they were functioning like a headless chicken, illustrated by the turn to Tarang Sharma. Whatever was going on in *BMJ*, the issue for the RIAT team was how to handle *BMJ*—whether to be nice and do as we were told in return for the prestige of a *BMJ* publication or to hang tough and to be prepared to walk away.

Round 9

After publication Tracey Brown, co-founder of AllTrials, leapt in: "When all trials are registered and results reported, it becomes possible for researchers to work out what data are available."

Iain Chalmers said, "Among pharmaceutical companies, GSK under its current management has led the way in promoting clinical trial transparency and provides a practical mechanism to make trial re-analyses possible. The reanalysis of Study 329 illustrates the knowledge dividends from the company's new policies and contrasts strikingly with the scientific misconduct that characterised the company's behaviour under previous management. Today's

GSK has shown moral and scientific leadership that puts to shame many in the academic community."

A year later Ben Goldacre was still stating in public that the Restored Study 329 had shown nothing new. Everything that needed to be known about this study had been known for many years.

BMJ, Ben Goldacre, Tracey Brown, Iain Chalmers, and GSK are all part of an AllTrials coalition.

The most important thing the RIAT study showed was that in assessing the integrity of reported research, we can have no confidence about harms without access to individual-level data. AllTrials does not see the need for access to the data. Its position of accepting the Clinical Study Report (CSR) as adequate to address trial integrity sells short those who have volunteered to participate in clinical trials for the benefit of others. AllTrials is fundamentally not interested in the harms a treatment may cause.

A year later in October 2016, Treximet, the combination of GSK's sumatriptan and naproxyn for migraine that Liz Loder had endorsed in 2014 just before its release featured in the Wall Street Journal as a shocking example of pharmaceutical industry price gouging. GSK had handed it over to Pernix who were charging $750 for 9 pills, when the combined cost of these two antediluvian pills bought separately was less than $5.

CHAPTER 11

Girl with a Headache

From the start to the finish of the Restoration of Study 329 the RIAT team logged over 250,000 email words, a huge proportion during the year dealing with the *BMJ*.

The single-screen remote desktop interface, the "periscope," that GSK offered was an enormous challenge. For Nardo, the efficacy analysis meant multiple spreadsheet tables opened simultaneously, with copying, pasting, cross-checking in a highly restrictive space. For Le Noury, they were even harder to manage, one page at a time. It required over a thousand hours to examine a third of the CRFs. Being unable to print, the team couldn't prepare packets to send to independent coders, make annotations or collate adverse events.

The Restoration created a unique situation. There is no other study in medicine that has two diametrically opposite representations in press simultaneously. The Keller paper could have been retracted but clearly won't be. But even if Keller's version had been retracted and "Restoring Study 329" stood alone, it would have been unique. There is no other article reporting the outcome of a clinical trial in medicine of an on-patent or recently on-patent pharmaceutical that comes with its data attached.

There is another equally important and exceptional feature of the Restored study. The abstract of a clinical trial will usually outline the methods used, the results found, and the conclusions drawn. It will not state:

> *Access to primary data from trials has important implications for both clinical practice and research, including that published conclusions about efficacy and safety should not be read as authoritative.*

BMJ and other journals often try to boil the lessons of a ten-page article down to a small box on the front page that has the take-home message—the drug works or doesn't, with this or that side effect. In the case of Restoring Study 329, the take-home message has nothing to do with the drug:

> *In the absence of access to primary data, misleading conclusions in publications of those trials can seem definitive.*
>
> *Access to primary data makes clear the many ways in which data can be analysed and represented, showing the importance of access to data and the value of reanalysis of trials.*
>
> *There are important implications for clinical practice, research, regulation of trials, licensing of drugs, and the sociology and philosophy of science*

And the final paragraph of the paper again has nothing to do with the drug and whether it works or is safe:

> *As with most scientific papers, Keller and colleagues convey an impression that "the data have spoken." This authoritative stance is possible only in the absence of access to the data. When the data become accessible to others, it becomes clear that scientific authorship is provisional rather than authoritative.*

There is nothing like this anywhere else in biomedicine. There are articles in the sociology of science and philosophy that make points like this, but no one trying to find out about their drug reads them. And there are few clinical trials that sociologists or philosophers engage with—faced with numbers, they turn tail.

But if you want to know about your drug or any drug you need to read this article—and not just read it, you need to play with the numbers and see what happens.

What follows is a précis of "Restoring Study 329"; the full copy is on the *study329.org* website. When you read the full copy, you will likely spot that the team has tried to echo the Keller version, down to repeating its wording in a number of places. The authors were frustrated in this by Elizabeth Loder, who just didn't seem to get what was going on

This playing with the ideas of the authority of science, authorship and ghost authorship gave Dr. Loder a blinding headache. It was not part of her understanding that the results of a trial might be legitimately authored and reauthored and in that sense there might be no truth. To the bitter end, she wanted the definitive truthful version of the study. But there is none.

The *study329.org* website invites you to join the club of 329 authors by posting suggested adjustments and conclusions on the website.

Restoring Study 329: Efficacy and harms of paroxetine and imipramine in the treatment of adolescent major depression: restoration of a randomised controlled trial

JOANNA LE NOURY, JOHN M NARDO, DAVID HEALY, JON JUREIDINI, MELISSA RAVEN, CATALIN TUFANARU, ELIA ABI-JAOUDE

ABSTRACT

Objectives: This is a reanalysis of GSK's Study 329 (published by Keller et al. in 2001), the primary objective of which was to compare the efficacy and safety of paroxetine and imipramine to placebo in the treatment of adolescents with unipolar major depression. The objective of this restoration under the Restoring Invisible and Abandoned Trials (RIAT) initiative was to see whether access to and reanalysis of a full dataset from a randomised controlled trial would have clinically relevant implications for evidence based medicine. **Design:** Double-blind randomised placebo-controlled trial. **Setting:** 12 North American academic psychiatry centres, from 20 April 1994 to 15 February 1998. Participants: 275 adolescents with major depression of at least 8 weeks in duration. Exclusion criteria included a range of comorbid psychiatric and medical disorders and suicidality. **Interventions:** Participants were randomised to 8 weeks double-blind treatment with paroxetine (20–40 mg), imipramine (200–300 mg), or placebo. **Main outcome measures:** The pre-specified primary efficacy variables were: change from baseline to the end of the 8-week acute treatment phase in total Hamilton Depression Scale (HAM-D) score; and the proportion of responders (HAM-D score ≤8 or ≥50% reduction in baseline HAM-D) at acute endpoint. Pre-specified secondary outcomes were (1) changes from baseline to endpoint in the following parameters: depression items in K-SADS-L; Clinical Global Impression; Autonomous Functioning Checklist; Self-Perception Profile; Sickness

Impact Scale, (2) predictors of response, (3) number of patients who relapse during the maintenance phase. Adverse experiences were to be coded and compared primarily using descriptive statistics. No coding dictionary was pre-specified. **Results:** The efficacy of paroxetine and imipramine was not statistically or clinically significantly different from placebo for any pre-specified primary or secondary efficacy outcome. HAM-D scores decreased by 10.73 [9.134 to 12.328], 8.95 [7.356, to 10.541] and 9.08 [7.450 to 10.708] points, least-squares mean [95% Confidence Interval], respectively, for the paroxetine, imipramine and placebo groups (p = 0.204). Clinically significant increases in harms were observed, including suicidal ideation and behaviour and other serious adverse events in the paroxetine group and cardiovascular problems in the imipramine group. More adverse events were identified with the RIAT than with the SKB/GSK methodology. **Conclusions:** Neither paroxetine nor high-dose imipramine demonstrated efficacy for major depression in adolescents, and there was an increase in harms with both drugs. Access to primary data from trials has important implications for both clinical practice and research, including that published conclusions about efficacy and safety should not be read as authoritative. The reanalysis of Study 329 illustrates the necessity of making primary trial data available to increase the rigour of the evidence base.

COMPETING INTERESTS

Healy has been and is an expert witness for plaintiffs in legal cases involving GSK's paroxetine, and for plaintiffs in actions involving other SSRIs. Jureidini has been an expert about documents obtained from GSK in a class action over study 329, and from Forest in relation to paediatric citalopram. Le Noury, Nardo, Raven, Tufanaru and Abi-Jaoude have nothing to declare.

BACKGROUND

In 2013 a RIAT initiative called for the publication of undisclosed outcomes in trials and the correction of misleading publications by independent groups if need be.

One misreported study was GSK's Study 329, led by Dr Martin Keller, a multicentre eight-week randomised controlled trial, followed by a six-month continuation phase, to compare the efficacy and safety of imipramine and paroxetine to placebo in the treatment of adolescents with depression. The study, published in 2001, has supported the use of antidepressants in adolescents since.

When asked if they intended to restore Study 329, GSK said no but following negotiation, they did provide access to the individual patient level data for Study 329 for reanalysis.

METHODS

The reanalysis used the Clinical Study Report (CSR), including Appendices A–G, along with approximately 77,000 pages of de-identified individual Case Report Forms (CRFs, Appendix H). All methods used are set out in the original 1994/1996 Study 329 protocol. Where the protocol was not specific, we chose standard methods that best presented the data.

The details about the centres, the patients, the randomisation procedure, sample size, medication compliance in the Keller paper were repeated here.

Primary efficacy variables were: change in total Hamilton Depression Scale (HAM-D) score and the proportion of *responders* at the end of the eight-week acute treatment phase (patients who had a 50% or greater reduction in the HAM-D or a HAM-D score equal to or less than 8).

There were a number of secondary efficacy variables also. Before and after breaking the blind, changes were made by the sponsors to these secondary outcomes. There is no document that provides a scientific rationale for these changes, which are therefore not reported.

The adverse event (AE) data come primarily from Appendix D. SKB/GSK used an Adverse Drug Events Coding System (ADECS) dictionary. We used the Medical Dictionary for Regulatory Activities (MedDRA) a system endorsed by the FDA and now used by GSK. MedDRA stays closer to the original description of events than ADECS; it codes suicidal events as 'suicidal ideation' or 'self-harm/attempted suicide' rather than the ADECS option of 'emotional lability'; similarly, aggression is more clearly flagged as 'aggressive events' rather than 'hostility'.

Most coding was straightforward. The vast majority of the verbatim terms simply mapped onto coding terms in MedDRA. Coding challenges stemmed from cases where there were significant adverse events, but GSK claimed the patients discontinued for lack of efficacy. There didn't have to be a patient narrative for such patients, where there had to be for patients discontinuing because of the adverse event. We have laid out all challenging coding decisions in Appendix 3.

The case report forms (Appendix H) were scrutinised for all AEs occurring during the acute, taper and follow-up phases. This identified additional events not recorded in Appendix D. It also led to recoding of a number of the reasons for discontinuation. All new adverse events and reasons for changing discontinuation category are recorded in Appendix 2. We did not undertake statistical tests of the harms data.

RESULTS

The efficacy of paroxetine and imipramine was not statistically or clinically significant compared to placebo for any primary or secondary outcome.

FIGURE 2: DOES PAROXETINE WORK?

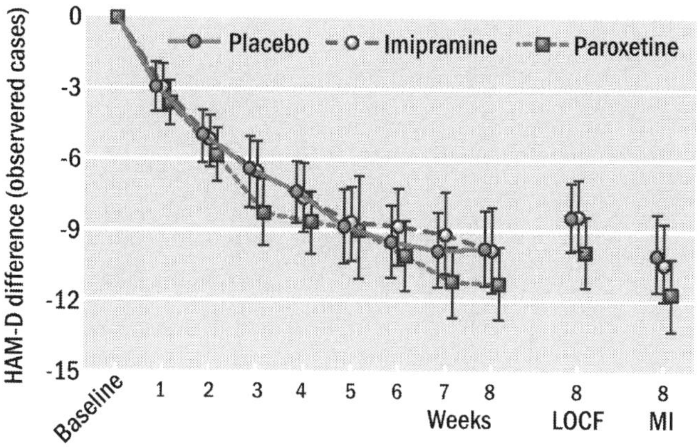

HARMS

TABLE 5: ADVERSE EVENTS

	Paroxetine (n = 93)		Imipramine (n = 95)		Placebo (n = 87)	
Adverse Event	**Keller***	**RIAT**	**Keller***	**RIAT**	**Keller***	**RIAT**
Cardiovascular	5	44	42	130	6	32
Gastro-intestinal	84	112	106	147	61	79
Psychiatric	—	103	—	63	—	24
Respiratory	33	42	27	22	37	39
Nervous system	115	101	135	114	65	77
Other	28	79	30	76	38	79
Total	265	481	340	552	207	330

TABLE 7: SERIOUS ADVERSE EVENTS

System	Paroxetine (n = 93)	Imipramine (n = 95)	Placebo (n = 87)
Cardiovascular	1	4	0
Gastro-intestinal	25	20	4
Psychiatric	32	4	5
Respiratory	2	1	4
Neurological	7	13	7
Other	10	21	12
Total	70	50	25

DISCUSSION

In our analysis of Study 329 neither paroxetine nor imipramine worked for major depression in adolescents. There was a clinically significant increase in harms with both drugs. This analysis contrasts with both the Keller article and GSK's Clinical Study Report.

The difference stems from keeping faith with the protocol methodology and its designation of primary and secondary outcome variables. Keller and GSK departed from the protocol by performing pairwise comparisons of two of the three groups when the omnibus ANOVA showed no significance in either the continuous or dichotomous variables. They also reported four other variables as significant that had been unmentioned in the protocol or its amendments, without any acknowledgment that these measures were introduced post hoc. This contravened provision II of Appendix B, Administrative Matters, according to which any changes to the study protocol were required to be filed as amendments/modifications.

With regard to adverse events, there were large differences between the data analysed by us, those summarised in the CSR, and those reported in Keller et al. These differences arise from inadequate and incomplete entry of data from CRFs to summary data sheets in the CSR, the ADECS coding system used by SKB/GSK, and the reporting of these data sheets in Keller et al.

One reason why Keller's figures differ from ours is because Keller et al. only presented data for adverse events reported for 5% of patients or more. They also differ because Keller did not report a category of psychiatric adverse events, but instead grouped psychiatric events together with 'dizziness' and 'headache' under nervous system. Since dizziness is more likely to be attributable to 'cardiovascular' while headaches are not psychiatric, we did not group them together with psychiatric adverse events. The effect of this change was to unmask a clinically important difference in psychiatric adverse event profiles between paroxetine and placebo.

There was a major difference between the frequency of suicidal thinking and events reported by Keller et al, and the frequency documented in the Clinical Study Report. Our CRF review added even more cases.

The coding for suicidal and self-injurious behaviours is fully detailed in RIAT Appendix 3.

Our reanalysis of study 329 revealed several ways in which the analysis and presentation of safety data can influence the apparent safety of a drug (see Box 2).

BOX 2. BARRIERS TO ACCURATE REPORTING OF HARMS

1. **Use of an idiosyncratic coding system**

   The term 'emotional lability' from SKB's ADECS masked discrepancies in suicidal behaviour between paroxetine and placebo.

2. **Failure to transcribe all adverse events from the clinical record to the adverse event database**

   Our review of Case Report Forms disclosed significant under-recording of adverse events.

3. **Filtering data on adverse events through statistical techniques**

Keller et al. and GSK ignored unfavourable harms data on the grounds that the difference between paroxetine and placebo was not statistically significant. Testing for statistical significance is most appropriately undertaken for efficacy measures. We have not undertaken statistical tests for harms, since we know of no valid way of interpreting them. To get away from a sterile statistically significant or not-significant presentation of evidence, we opted to present all the evidence and allow readers their own interpretation in RIAT Appendix 2 and related worksheets for those interested, and we welcome other analyses.

4. **Restriction of reporting to events that occurred above a given frequency in any one group**

The Keller paper reported only adverse events that occurred in more than 5% of patients. We report all adverse events. These are available in RIAT Appendix 2.

5. **Coding an event under different headings for different patients (dilution)**

An adverse effect like agitation may be coded under agitation, anxiety, nervousness, hyperkinesis and emotional lability. In this way, a problem occurring at a 10% rate could vanish if none of subheadings reached a threshold rate of 5%.

Aside from making all data available so that others can scrutinize it, one way to compensate for this possibility is to present all the data in broader groups. MedDRA offers the following higher levels: psychiatric; cardiovascular; gastrointestinal; respiratory; and other.

6. Grouping of adverse events

Even when presented in broader system groups, grouping common and benign symptoms with serious ones can mask safety issues. For example, Keller grouped dizziness and headaches with psychiatric adverse events under a 'nervous system' heading. This diluted the difference in psychiatric side effects between paroxetine, imipramine and placebo.

We have reported dizziness under 'cardiovascular' and headache under 'nervous system'. There may be better categorisations. In Appendix 2, we have listed all events coded under each heading and we invite others to explore alternative higher level grouping.

7. Rating severity

In addition to coding adverse events, investigators rate them for severity. If no attempt is made to take severity into account, readers may get the impression that there was an equal adverse event burden in each arm, when in fact all events in one arm might be severe and enduring while those in the other might be mild and transient.

One way to manage this is to look specifically at those patients who drop out because of adverse events. Another is to select adverse events coded as severe omitting those coded as mild or moderate. We used both approaches.

8. Relatedness coding

Judgements by investigators as to whether an adverse event is related to the drug can discount the importance of an effect. It also became clear that the blind had been broken in several cases before relatedness was adjudicated. For instance, it is documented in the Clinical Study Report (p. 279) that an investigator, knowing the patient was on placebo, declared that a suicidal event was 'definitely related to treatment', on the grounds that 'the worsening of depression and suicidal thought were life threatening and definitely related to study medication [known to be placebo] in that there was a lack of effect'. Of the 11 patients with serious adverse events on paroxetine compared to two on placebo reported in the Keller paper, only one 'was considered by the treating investigator to be related to paroxetine treatment', dismissing the difference between the paroxetine and placebo groups for serious adverse events.

9. **Masking effects of concomitant medication**

Other medications will obscure differences between active drug and placebo and may be significant in trials of treatments such as statins, where patients are on multiple medications.

We compared the adverse events in those on versus those not on other medication—see Appendix 2. There are other angles in this data that could be explored, such as the effects of withdrawal of concomitant medication as the spreadsheets offer the day of onset of adverse events and the dates of starting or stopping any concomitant medication. Another option is to look for prescribing cascades triggered by adverse events related to study medication.

10. **The effects of medication withdrawal**

The protocol included a 7–17 day taper phase. The original paper did not analyse these data. We have done. They point to dependence on and withdrawal from paroxetine.

CONCLUSION

Contrary to the Keller et al. article, Study 329 showed no advantage for paroxetine or imipramine over placebo in adolescent depression. There were increases in severe and suicide related adverse events in the paroxetine and imipramine arms. Some of the problems only became apparent when the data were made available for reanalysis. Researchers, clinicians and regulators should mandate access to data.

As with most scientific papers, Keller et al. conveys an impression that 'the data have spoken'. This authoritative stance is only possible in the absence of access to the data. When the data become accessible to others, it becomes clear that scientific authorship is provisional rather than authoritative.

REFERENCES 27

See references and the complete study on www.study329.org

CHAPTER 13

Emotionally Labile Girl

The suicidal cases in Study 329 were at the heart of the Department of Justice's case against GSK.[145] There were differing views as to how many cases there were—FDA's view, GSK's view, the RIAT view, and events that have come to light since.

In its approvable letter in October 2002 to GSK, the FDA asked for additional information about patients in the studies who had experienced adverse events and who had withdrawn prematurely, as well as why GSK used the term emotional lability to describe the five patients who attempted to commit suicide or exhibited other self-injurious behaviour.

In May 2003, GSK provided the additional safety data. It told FDA there was no statistically significant difference in suicidality between placebo and Paxil in all the Paxil paediatric depression studies cumulatively. But there were many more suicidal events on Paxil, and the difference between these events on Paxil versus events on placebo became statistically significant if the first 30 days after therapy were included in the analysis.

GSK also admitted at this point that there were four more possible events on Paxil patients in Study 329. The FDA then identified another event not among the 11 serious adverse events listed in the Keller paper. Thus, altogether, 10 of the 93 Paxil patients in Study 329 experienced a possibly suicidal event, compared to 1 of the 87 patients on a placebo—a different picture of Paxil's paediatric safety profile than the one painted by Keller and co-authors, which listed 5 possibly suicidal events on Paxil, brushed those off as unrelated to Paxil, and concluded that treating children with Paxil was safe.

But there were even more events than FDA or GSK listed.

Table A: Suicidal and self-injurious behaviours in Study 329

	Paroxetine Patients (events)	Imipramine Patients (events)	Placebo Patients (events)
Keller et al.	5	3	1
GSK Acute	7	3	1
GSK Continuation & Taper	2 previous + 2 new	1	1
GSK Total	9	4	2
FDA	10	4	2
RIAT Acute & Taper	11 (14)	4 (6)	2
RIAT Continuation	1 previous + 1 new	1	2
RIAT Total	12 (15)	5 (7) 4 definite 1 possible	4 2 definite 2 possible

Table B: Suicidal cases in Study 329

Case	Keller	GSK	FDA	RIAT	Appendix (pages)		Clinical Study Report (pages)	
					D	G	Acute	Contin.
1		X	X	X	125	167		173
2	X	X	X	X	28, 127	341	283	
3	X	X	X	X	28, 131	511	288	177
4	X	X	X	X	28, 132	553	289	
5		X	X	X	28, 132	607		
6	X	X	X	X	28, 143	1074	294	
7				X	11, 144	1082		
8	X	X	X	X	25, 29, 124	29, 277	107, 272	
9		X	X	X	28, 142	142	272, 292	
10			X	X		257	281	
11		X	X	X		28, 137	782-83	500
12				X		28	442	272, 285

Case Number and Patient IDs

Case	Patient ID
1	329.002.00058
2	329.002.00245
3	329.003.00250
4	329.003.00313
5	329.004.00015
6	329.006.00038
7	329.006.00039
8	329.001.00065
9	329.005.00333
10	329.002.00106
11	329.005.00011
12	329.005.00089

Coding and its challenges

You will likely disagree with us on some of the points below. This is as it should be. Before revealing the cases on which we might disagree, it is worth reviewing the issues coding throws up.

Coding involves a balance between coding flat with no presuppositions or applying expertise. A layperson is likely better at coding flat. In terms of expertise, specialist knowledge and looking at the context can add important dimensions but can also mislead.

Case #7 (ID 329.006.00039) highlights these points. Taking a lay coder approach, coding superficial scratches as trauma makes sense. Taking an expert approach might lead to the same coding as "we know" that many of these "gestures" in adolescents are not "truly" suicidal.

The expert "we know that this one is not truly suicidal" needs to be resisted for a few reasons. First we have to resist because the FDA insists on it—it insisted, for instance, that case 00015, which is self-mutilation, but where the clinician insisted it was not suicidal, has to be included in the self-harm/suicidal group.

There is a reason behind this. A lot of completed suicides are not intended—as when people playing with thoughts of suicide, kneel down with a noose around their neck and lean forward, not realizing that they can lose consciousness this way, and once they do, they strangle themselves. Gestures can kill, and if SSRIs increase the rate of gestures, they may increase death rates.

Equally, in clinical practice, there are cases where there is real planning and lethal effort but the person survives and when asked afterwards can offer no reason for why they did what they did. Most liaison services regularly see cases like this, who might be extraverts, or what were once called alexithymics, but the point is one cannot just rely on stated intent.

Finally, coding all "trivial" events should increase the noise in the system, and other things being equal, this should work to the drug's advantage, as it will hide true signals. So if a company wants to hide problems, a better strategy in the case of blind coding is to overcode suicidality rather than undercode it. It is highly likely that within these clinical trial databases there are a number of other suicide-related events coded under headings such as thinking abnormally or nightmares.

Appendix 3 in the published paper includes a Table C, which provides details of possibly more cases and exactly where in the 329 haystack each of these needles can be found.

Case #7 (ID: 329.006.00039)

The events in this case were described as "superficial scratches." GSK coded this as trauma. There were two cases of superficial lacerations coded as trauma—case #7 (superficial scratches) and case 00197 (superficial laceration to the scalp). The RIAT authors coded both of these blind and coded both as suicidal. Case 00197 is a placebo case from the continuation phase.

The context partly influenced the choice of suicidality over trauma as the right coding option. There were 18 other trauma cases, 12 on placebo, 5 on paroxetine and 1 on imipramine (spreadsheet available on *study329.org*). All involved fractures or sprains rather than lacerations and were coded as trauma. Three of these cases had serious adverse event (SAE) narratives in the Clinical Study Report. These give a good "feel" for cases that both SmithKline and RIAT coded as trauma.

In contrast, there were two cases of superficial scratches on paroxetine—cases #7 and #4 (ID: 329.003.00313). In case #4, SmithKline coded superficial scratches as emotional lability. Case #4 generated an SAE narrative, whereas #7 did not. The narrative version of the verbatim term superficial scratches in case #4 was as follows:

He has cut himself in response to the voice on three occasions in the past six days. On the back of his hand he has carved a cross with small adorning cuts. On his forearms he has made 10–15 cuts each about six inches long. On his upper arm are three additional cuts.

Clearly this cannot be trauma, and GSK coded it as emotional lability.

There was no comparable narrative for 00039, but the adverse event sheet shows that the superficial scratches happened over ten days and involved multiple events happening continuously. This is not consistent with trauma.

In #7, the HAM-D and Kiddie-SADS rating scales also recorded increased suicidal ideation/gestures during this period and a later episode of suicidal ideation at week six, and at week six aggravated depression was also listed as an adverse event in the CRF but did not make its way into the CSR.

The main use of the raw data (the CRF) in this case was to ensure that it contained nothing that would support a trauma coding. If there had been any indication of trauma other than its use as a verbatim term, the RIAT team would have coded as trauma.

Based on the above, RIAT recoded case #7 as "suicidal event—self-harm" and added "suicidal ideation" (at week six).

In contrast, the placebo case 00197 shows zero ratings on suicide items.

Case #12 (ID: 329.005.00089)

This paroxetine patient was coded as euphoria by SmithKline. The narrative states that, starting at week four, her "behavioral symptoms worsened over the next two weeks through to completion of week eight of the study." The patient reported increased feelings of elation and expansive mood. There was also a decreased need for sleep, increased energy and inflated self-esteem. Other symptoms included accelerated speech, flight of ideas and motor hyperactivity. The school reported "impulsive and sexually provocative behaviour."

This is all consistent with bipolar disorder, to which there are a number of steers in the manuscript; therefore GSK's coding of euphoria seems reasonable.

In this case, it would be appropriate to code grandiosity, impulsive behaviour, disinhibition, expansive mood, decreased need for sleep, increased energy, inflated self-esteem, accelerated speech, flight of ideas, motor hyperactivity, sexually provocative behaviour, agitation and suicidal behaviour. All that is coded is euphoria and insomnia.

Euphoria is listed in Appendix D page 130 as starting on April 4, as severe and as leading to the drug being stopped. It is classed as serious because it led to hospitalization.

But the narrative also contains the following: On May 2, eight weeks after entering the study, "the patient became agitated and said she would kill herself following threats of punishment from her mother to control her behaviour. The patient was deemed at risk to herself and was brought to the crisis service. She was hospitalized… and the decision was made she would not enter the continuation phase."

The rating scales at this point also record significant suicidality, where there had been none before.

This patient had four different CRFs. There was as much as 40 pages in the difference between the number of pages in different versions. A week before the event, one version of the CRF records the patient as being down-titrated from four paroxetine tablets to three per day, but another version of the CRF removes this down-titration.

In this case, the study monitors also made an additional note recording a series of significant discrepancies between the SAE narrative in the clinical study report and the CRF(s).

Case #10 (ID: 329.002.00106)

On day 51, having apparently stopped her medication three days before, this patient threatened suicide in the course of what was reported to be an argument with her mother. She was hospitalized for two weeks. Her HAM-D scores prior to the event reveal nothing. She was discontinued from the study, and there was no further assessment or follow up.

In Appendix D, the original verbatim term was "psychiatric hospitalization," but this was scratched out and replaced with "oppositional defiant disorder," which was then coded in ADECS as hostility.

The query log raises the possibility that stopping the drug was part of an oppositional defiant disorder adverse event, which apparently went on for two days, according to the adverse event section.

For several reasons, this case looks most likely to be the one that the Department of Justice complaint cited above mentions as an extra suicidal event picked up by FDA.

It is suicidal event; whether or not it is the FDA extra event is a moot point.

Taper patients

Two other patients, Case #1 (ID: 329.002.00058) and Case #3 (ID: 329.003.00250), are of interest. In both cases the event happened during taper according to RIAT, or continuation according to GSK.

Case #1 (ID: 329.002.00058)

GSK agrees that this case was a suicidal event but listed it in the continuation phase. Anyone skimming the serious adverse event narrative will likely agree with GSK, as the event appears to happen in the middle of the continuation phase.

But the date for the end of the continuation phase in this narrative is the notional, not the actual, end of the phase. Some reviewer may have made an innocent mistake here.

In fact this patient had stopped the drug three days before the overdose, then overdosed and was discontinued completely from the study—three months before an independent assessor might have innocently thought they stopped taking the drug. On this basis RIAT has put the case into taper.

For GSK, in contrast, it seems once you enter continuation, you are no longer acute, whereas the RIAT authors have opted for a deferred taper phase in people who go into continuation.

There is a real question about whether it is correct to treat all acute patients equally, in which case a purist will do what RIAT did. Others might accept that all acute patients cannot be treated equally—some have tapers and some do not.

There is no settled view on this issue. It may be an issue the field does not know exists.

There are other notable things about case Case #1. For example, most pages where the adverse events section should be are missing—but fortunately the page with the intentional overdose is present.

Case #3 (ID: 329.003.00250)

This case has suicide attempts in the acute phase and what GSK calls the continuation phase. The company recognizes both events, and codes both as emotional lability.

For the second event, the patient is poised between acute and continuation phases. They appear to run out of medication. The medication is tapered from paroxetine 40 mg to 30 mg, at which point the overdose happens and the patient is discontinued.

There has been no continuation phase documentation filled. After the overdose, the first continuation phase pages are filled, noting that this patient is being discontinued because of an overdose.

GSK regards the patient as having entered the continuation phase because of this, although not a single continuation phase tablet is taken.

This is a patient on the cliff between the acute and continuation phases. One third of the patients in this study disappear into this crevasse.

Placing this patient in taper rather than continuation makes no difference to the number of suicidal patients, but it makes a difference to the number of events. This again is a matter of interpretation. We think the appropriate way forward is to note the ambiguity—which is not fully clear in the appendix.

Case #5 (ID: 329.004.00015)

SmithKline codes self-mutilation in this case as emotional lability. The RIAT authors coded it as suicide attempt. SmithKline has another event in the continuation phase—suicidal ideation. The restoration authors agree.

We note a further possible suicidal ideation in the acute phase. The HAM-D score a few days after the suicide attempt is a 3—this may just refer to the gesture earlier that week or to accompanying suicidal ideation. The Kiddie-SADS covering the same period scores on the self-mutilation options and on the suicidal ideation option, while insisting that the self- mutilation was not suicidal.

Reviewing this CRF is unhelpful. Every problem feels minimized except for log notes about the patient's weight. The patient later drops out of the study.

When patients drop out of a study for serious adverse events, companies are obliged to write a narrative that often sheds more light on what has been happening. There are 17 patients in Study 329 on whom SmithKline wrote such narratives—11 paroxetine, 5 imipramine and 1 placebo patient in the acute phase and more in the continuation phase. Case #5 is not among them.

There are other cases in the acute and continuation phases with serious events who do not drop out. In such cases, a company is not obliged to write narratives but often does.

Case #5 has events that many would call serious but these are coded as mild—no narratives were written.

When a patient drops out of the study, the company must code the reason for withdrawal. In this case you might have expected "adverse events" or "lack of efficacy." But SmithKline's stated reason is "other," and it cites a clash between school and this research study.

New cases

In response to queries from a movie scriptwriter, Healy and Le Noury were reviewing their files two years after publication and realized they had missed a raft of cases.

One of the oddities of Study 329 was that all the suicidal cases came from centres 1 through 6 with none from 7 through 12. These centres had been brought on stream later, so there were fewer cases but still... none!

Then we came across an email from Karen Tennenbaum to SmithKline Beecham on April 5 1996 about case 329.009.00201—from the Dallas centre, where Graham Emslie was based, one of the centres from which there had been no other reports.

This patient:

> *Apparently became manic and had a gun. He was taken to the hospital where—blank—was attending him. Blank—called SB to determine the blinded medication so the patient could be appropriately treated.*

The patient was taking Paxil. He was coded as intercurrent illness. This means that SB decided he had bipolar disorder or paranoia or whatever and that this was the source of the problems rather than he had a reaction to their drug. He was not filed under lack of efficacy or adverse event and there was no patient narrative to tell us more.

There were several other cases coded this way—including another from Dallas. This looks like a very deliberate hiding of treatment induced problems.

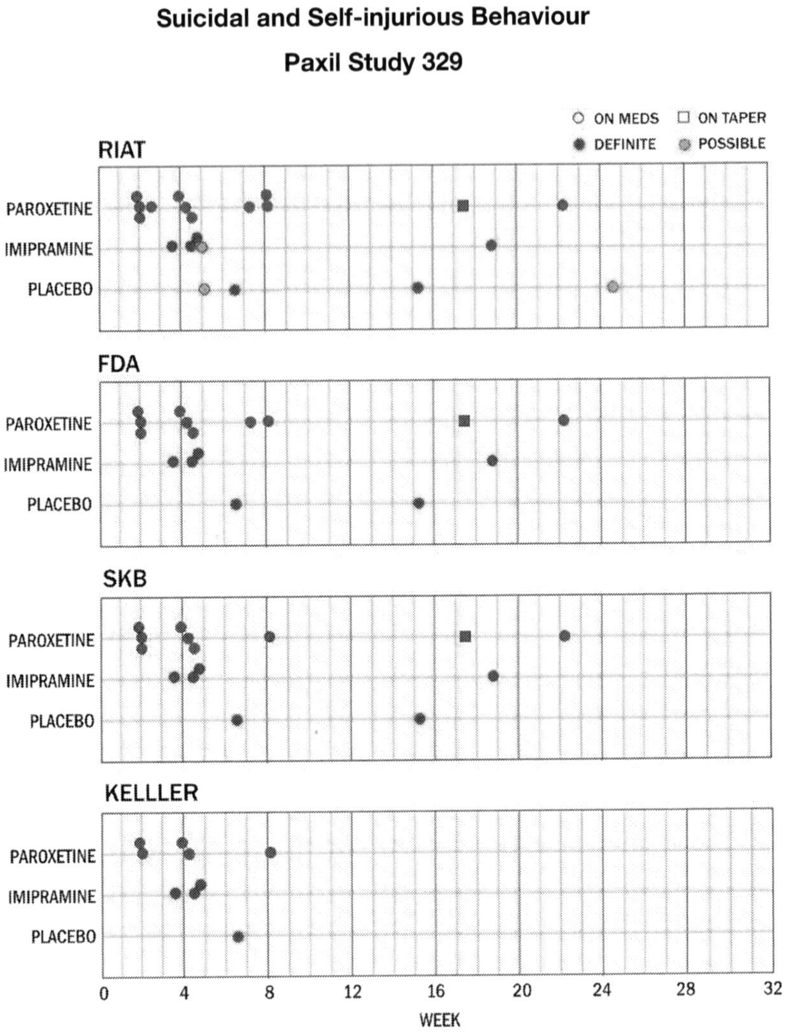
Suicidal and Self-injurious Behaviour
Paxil Study 329
ON MEDS
ON TAPER
DEFINITE
POSSIBLE
RIAT
PAROXETINE
IMIPRAMINE
PLACEBO
FDA
PAROXETINE
IMIPRAMINE
PLACEBO
SKB
PAROXETINE
IMIPRAMINE
PLACEBO
KELLLER
PAROXETINE
IMIPRAMINE
PLACEBO
0
4
8
12
16
20
24
28
32
WEEK

CHAPTER 13

Research Parasites

Almost the minute "Restoring Study 329" went live, GSK issued a written statement saying that it had cooperated fully with the *BMJ* reanalysis and that the company now recognizes that "there is an increased risk of suicidality in pediatric and adolescent patients given antidepressants like paroxetine."

It looked a safer bet tactically for Martin Keller and his colleagues to remain silent, but much to our surprise, they also broke cover. Keller contacted The Chronicle to insist that the 2001 results faithfully represented the best effort of the authors at the time, and that any misrepresentation of his article to help sell Paxil was the responsibility of Glaxo.

"Nothing was ever pinned on any of us," despite various trials and investigations, he said. "And when I say that, I'm not telling you we're like the great escape artists, that we're Houdinis and we did something wrong and we got away with the crime of the century. Don't you think if there was really something wrong, some university or agency or something would have pinned something on us?"[146]

In what he described as his first effort to speak publicly about the matter, Keller said his critics also have financial and professional motives for amplifying criticisms, including lawyers representing Paxil plaintiffs and professors seeking their own records of journal publication. He made it clear that he and his co-authors would be responding in more detail.

BMJ has a Rapid Response section where comments on an article can be submitted. There were many comments in the case of Study 329, most of them anodyne. The most interesting came from David Linden of Cardiff:

> *If one sticks to the MedDRA primary system organ class (SOC), one obtains different results for the adverse events from those presented in*

> *Table 5 of the paper. For example, psychiatric adverse events decrease (from 103 to 57 in the paroxetine group, from 63 to 37 in the imipramine group and from 24 to 13 in the placebo group, (see Table below), largely because of the reclassification of akathisia and somnolence into nervous system disorders. Conversely, the nervous systems disorders increase (from 101 to 160 in the paroxetine group, from 114 to 178 in the imipramine group and from 77 to 91 in the placebo group). Although, looking at the verbatim terms in the spreadsheet, it is understandable why the authors classified akathisia as "psychiatric;" the case is less clear for somnolence. In general, I would be interested in the authors' comment on the scope for interpretation left open by their approach.*[147]

This was the only response that demonstrated a full understanding that the Restoration of Study 329 was about authorship. Scientific articles are authored, not delivered on tablets of stone from the top of a mountain; they can and should be contested.[148] Any reader can go in and play with the data the way David Linden did.

By January there had been no further reply from Keller. Documents that had come to light in depositions had made it clear there was a flurry of internal communication among the Keller team in June 2004—around the time New York State filed its fraud action.

> *I am extremely concerned that leaving us vulnerable to the wolves is not a major or even minor concern to our "partners" [GSK]... We are not without leverage if we are dissatisfied and want to play a little hardball of our own.*
>
> *A critical issue will be whether working together we are able to explain in detail what is different here than in 329, about 329 and in the presentation about the other two studies, so that it is 100% clear in this paper that there is no way to read it and think that 329 is being criticized and that it was not written with complete integrity and accuracy given the data we had and should have had as investigators... otherwise*

> *we could look foolish, naïve, incompetent or " biased " to present things in a way that was favourable to SK, disregarding our responsibility to the proper scientific method, to the public, children and their families.*

In the meantime, "Restoring Study 329" kicked off a debate about data access. The most extraordinary contribution to this debate came from Jeffrey Drazen, the editor of the New England Journal of Medicine, in January 2016. Drazen, who opposes data access, wrote:

> *The aerial view of the concept of data sharing is beautiful. What could be better than having high-quality information carefully re-examined for the possibility that new nuggets of useful data are lying there, previously unseen? The potential for leveraging existing results for even more benefit pays appropriate increased tribute to the patients who put themselves at risk to generate the data. The moral imperative to honor their collective sacrifice is the trump card that takes this trick...*
>
> *A second concern held by some is that a new class of research person will emerge—people who had nothing to do with the design and execution of the study but use another group's data for their own ends, possibly stealing from the research productivity planned by the data gatherers, or even use the data to try to disprove what the original investigators had posited. There is concern among some front-line researchers that the system will be taken over by what some researchers have characterized as "research parasites."*[149]

The term research parasite was quickly hashtagged and became an academic social media hit. Lots of people identified as research parasites, perhaps just to annoy Drazen.

Nothing was pinned on us

Then on January 19, Keller and nine of his co-authors—Birmaher, Carlson, Clarke, Emslie, Koplewicz, Kutcher, Ryan, Sack and Strober—responded, alleging a lack of detailed methodology, bias within the RIAT team, lack of blind ratings in relation to harms and failure to consider the available knowledge regarding paediatric depression from 24 years ago:

1. *Authors of "Restoring Study 329" evidenced both bias and a lack of blind ratings. In a recent article about "Restoring Study 329" in the Chronicle of Higher Education, Dr. Jureidini is quoted as saying: "We don't think we've done the definitive analysis. It's not something that can be done absolutely objectively, particularly the interpretation of harms. We can't protect ourselves completely from our own biases."*

   Biases are a serious consideration for Restoring Study 329 because Dr. Jureidini, as he declares in a footnote on the subject of "Competing interests," served as an expert witness for plaintiff's lawyers in legal suits against GSK related to Study 329. In that work Dr. Jureidini would have studied all available data looking at both efficacy and suicidal side effects, using many different approaches to best capture any potential harms.

2. *The "restoring invisible and abandoned trials" (RIAT) approach to re-analyzing published studies may provide general guidelines, but we could not find publications or available working RIAT documents on detailed protocols. Lack of detailed methodology is a serious concern because there is general consensus in the field that there is not, nor never will be, a single correct approach to re-analysis. Small differences in analysis frequently make big differences in statistical results and conclusions.*

3. *"Restoring Study 329" did not consider available knowledge 24 years ago, when Paroxetine 329 was developed and performed. Clinical research methodology has evolved considerably in the past two decades. These aspects are addressed in comments by established investigators not involved in Paroxetine 329. For example, Referring to "Restoring Study 329" as reported in Psychiatric News Alert [4] Mark Olfson said, "However, the new re-analysis does not alter the totality of clinical trial evidence that continues to support the safety and efficacy of SSRIs for adolescent depression." And Daniel Pine said, "We have known for some time that antidepressant medications have both significant benefits for some children as well as significant risks for other children. This new analysis really does nothing to change this knowledge, and provides no new insights into what we have known about these medications for the past few years."*[150]

They defended how they handled the analysis of the efficacy data, reiterating that in the abstract of the original paper "we stated, 'Conclusions: Paroxetine is generally well tolerated and effective for major depression in adolescents.' In this sample and with the state of knowledge at the time, it was justified and appropriate."

They again claimed additional secondary outcome measures were put in place mid-trial, however, despite being provided with ample opportunity to provide documentary evidence to this effect, to date no evidence has ever been provided to support this:

> *In the interval from when we planned the study to when we approached the data analysis phase, but prior to the blind being broken, the academic authors, not the sponsor, added several additional measures of depression as secondary outcomes. We did so because the field of pediatric-age depression had reached a consensus that the Hamilton Depression Rating Scale (our primary outcome measure) had significant limitations in assessing mood disturbance in younger patients. Taking this into consideration, and in advance of breaking the blind, we added secondary outcome measures agreed upon by all authors of the paper. We found statistically significant indications of efficacy in these measures. These secondary outcomes were clearly reported as separate from the negative primary outcomes.*
>
> *Thus, the authors of* "BMJ—Restoring Study 329" *were incorrect in stating that:*
>
> > *Both before and after breaking the blind, however, the sponsors made changes to the secondary outcomes as previously detailed. We could not find any document that provided any scientific rationale for these post hoc changes and the outcomes are therefore not reported in this paper.*
>
> *Rather, secondary outcomes were decided by the authors prior to the blind being broken. Secondary outcome measures are frequently, and appropriately, included in study reports even when the primary measures do not reach statistical significance. The authors of "Restoring Study*

> *329" state "there were no discrepancies between any of our analyses and those contained in the CSR [clinical study report]." The disagreement on treatment outcomes rests on this arbitrary and non-blind dismissal of our secondary outcome measures.*

They critiqued the RIAT analysis of the adverse events data and specifically the issue of suicidality:

> *We emphatically disagree with the "Restoring Study 329" position that statistics are not useful in understanding adverse side effects and that each individual reader should decide for herself when a difference in rates of adverse side effects is meaningful. Statistics offer several approaches to the question of when is there a meaningful difference in the side effect rates between different treatments.*
>
> *Specific methodology problems in the re-analysis of the "harm" data are as follows:*
>
> 1. *The authors choose a non-random subsample of 85 subjects who were withdrawn from the study plus 8 subjects whom the authors labeled "suicidal" based on their inspection of the data;*
> 2. *A different instrument was utilized to re-score the harm effects, and only one of the authors was trained in the scoring of the instrument;*
> 3. *Some side effects were arbitrarily interpreted (e.g., upper respiratory symptoms were labeled as "dystonia" and emotional lability labeled as "suicidality");*
> 4. *In the original paper, side effects were analyzed only during the acute phase, but in the re-analysis, the authors analyzed them during the acute phase, as well as the tapering and follow up phases of the study; and*
> 5. *In the original study patients were interviewed face-to-face, whereas the re-analysis was based only on the interpretation of the data; and*

6. *Importantly, the two authors were not blind to patients' randomization status.*

Suicidal ideation and attempts

1. *Our field's understanding of how to approach analysis of suicidal ideation, suicide attempts, and completed suicide has advanced enormously since publication of study 329.*
2. *Two definitive re-analyses of the suicidality with antidepressants in adolescents include:*
3. *The 2003 FDA re-analysis of all RCT data of SSRI studies in youth for all indications.[6] In the FDA analysis the average risk ratio for SSRI versus placebo treated subjects was 1.96 (CI: 1.28-2.98). Considered separately, Study 329 did not reach statistical significance for increased suicidality (CI: 0.42-33.21).*
4. *The methodologically superior re-analysis by Bridge and colleagues also found that in study 329 there was no significant risk difference between paroxetine and placebo.*

Paroxetine treatment in youth does not appear to significantly differ from other SSRIs in the risk of suicidal ideation or attempts and whether SSRIs increase or decrease completed suicide remains an open question.

They concluded:

We strongly support efforts to make anonymized raw data from scientific studies available for re-analysis. The validity of "Restoring 329," however, is doubtful because of author bias and substantial problems with RIAT methodology. To describe Paroxetine 329 as "misreported" is pejorative and wrong based on both state-of-the-art research methods 24 years ago, and retrospectively from the standpoint of current best practices.

The Keller response gave Peter Doshi and Tom Jefferson an opportunity to explain more about RIAT:

RIAT is a conceptual framework for bringing corrective action to the scientific literature by publishing unpublished trials and re-publishing published-but-misreported clinical trials. The 2015 publication by Le Noury et al. used the RIAT framework to republish Study 329. The basis for this was the misreporting of the study by Keller et al. in their 2001 publication in JAACAP*. This publication was a key piece of evidence in the U.S. Department of Justice criminal lawsuit against GlaxoSmith-Kline which ultimately settled for U.S. $3 billion in 2012. Other researchers have used the RIAT framework to publish an unpublished trial on colorectal surgery.*

The RIAT declaration outlines a number of steps that "restorative authors" (here, Le Noury et al.) should use to enable an ethical primary publication of a clinical trial. A key one is that RIAT papers must report the clinical trial according to the original protocol of the original trial. Any analyses conducted that were not pre-specified in the original protocol must be clearly marked as such. (We wrote: "RIAT analyses should follow the analyses specified in the protocol [including any specified in amendments]. Any other analyses are discouraged, but if done must be clearly noted as exploratory and not pre-specified. At the same time, RIAT authors may wish to critically appraise the trials they report. This can be useful, but the critique should be clearly identifiable and placed in the discussion section.")

PD [Peter Doshi] served as one of the formal peer reviewers for the Le Noury paper and as far as he can tell, the authors followed this guidance.

We and our co-authors specifically intended RIAT to be a living concept, open to suggestions for improvement. While Keller et al. express concern over a lack of "detailed methodology" for RIAT, they do not cite the RIAT declaration nor mention any details of what is actually lacking in the current process. We invite them to read the RIAT declaration.[151]

The RIAT team also responded to Keller and his colleagues:

While there was uncertainty twenty-four years ago about the appropriate rating scale to use in pediatric depression trials, there were serious methodological problems in the conduct and reporting of Study 329 that have nothing to do with that uncertainty. Instead, in their reporting of efficacy in Study 329, and their defence of it, Keller and colleagues have asked that the field suspend many widely held tenets about clinical trial analysis, by asking us to do the following:

- *Accept that the a priori protocol is not binding, and that changes can be made to the outcome variables while the study is ongoing, without amending the protocol with the IRB or documenting the rationale for the change*
- *Ignore the requirement to correct the threshold of significance for the analysis of multiple variables*
- *Ignore the requirement that when there are more than two groups, preliminary omnibus statistical analysis needs to be done prior to making any pairwise comparisons between groups—an integral part of the ANOVA analysis declared in the Study 329 protocol*
- *Allow the parametric analysis of rank-order, ordinal rating scales [CGI, HAM-D and K-SADS-L Depressed Mood Items] rather than the expected non-parametric methods specifically derived for this kind of data*
- *Allow 19 outcome measures to be added to the original eight at various times up to and after the breaking of the blind, purportedly according to an analytical plan "developed prior to opening of the blind" (In spite of multiple requests, neither GSK nor Keller and colleagues have ever produced this analytic plan, suggesting that either it does not exist, or that it contains information unsympathetic to their claims.)*
- *Accept the dismissal of protocol-specified secondary outcomes and the introduction of rogue variables on the grounds that "the Hamilton Depression Rating Scale (our primary outcome measure) had significant limitations in assessing mood disturbance in younger patients,"*

when none of the protocol-specified secondary outcome measures that they discarded were based on the HAM-D, and two of the rogue measures that they introduced were HAM-D measures

- *Accept the clinically dubious improvements in four of these rogue variables as evidence of efficacy. (Although these measures achieved statistical significance in the pre-defined eighth (final) week of the acute phase of the study, they did not do so in the weekly assessments over the previous seven weeks, a pattern unseen in any known antidepressant; we are working on another manuscript analysing Keller et al.'s rogue variables.)*
- *There was no ambiguity about the appropriateness of these methodological manoeuvres when Study 329 was conducted and reported. However, although some of these problems were obvious when the paper was first published, others were not apparent until we had access to the raw clinical data. This lack of transparency erodes confidence that RCTs will be conducted, analysed, and reported free from covert manipulation.*

Furthermore, Keller and colleagues also failed to report on the continuation phase of Study 329, even though that was a protocol-specified outcome. A report of this phase is almost ready for submission by us.

With regard to harms, Keller and colleagues are simply incorrect in many of their claims about our purported bias and lack of blind ratings.

First, our paper makes it clear that both coders in the re-analysis were blind to randomisation status.

Second, there was no "re-scoring." This odd choice of words raises doubts that Keller et al. have much expertise in analysing harms. We used a dictionary that adhered much more closely to the verbatim terms used by the face-to-face interviewers. The fact that Keller and colleagues say that we have labelled emotional lability as suicidality makes us wonder if they have seen the individual patient level data; it was the SKBs coders who came up with the term "emotional lability," not the face-to-face interviewers, whose verbatim terms were of suicidal thoughts and behaviour. Simply using the verbatim terms that the named authors or their colleagues had used when faced with these adolescents reveals a striking rate of suicidal events. To argue that our return to these verbatim terms was arbitrary is bizarre.

Third, we made it clear there is unavoidable uncertainty in coding, and we invited others to download the data we have made available and juggle it to see if they can improve on our categorisation of the data. In our correspondence with BMJ, *we made it clear that there are items that GSK could argue are more appropriately coded differently. We would be receptive to a rationale for alternate coding of certain items that is cogently argued rather than simply asserted, but our hunch is that a disinterested observer reviewing the coding as presented by GSK across all 1500 adverse effects in this study (or 2000+ if we include the continuation phase) would conclude that our efforts are a better representation of the data.*

Fourth, reading our paper makes it clear why we reviewed the clinical records of 93 subjects; these were the subjects who dropped out or became suicidal. Our claims about underreporting of adverse events stand independently of that non-random sub-sample.

With regard to suicidal ideation and attempts, Keller et al. refer to a re-analysis by Bridge and colleagues, which found that there was no significant difference in suicidality between paroxetine and placebo. But Bridge et al. relied on Keller et al.'s misleading 2001 report.

With regard to bias, our point was that the best protection against bias is rigorous adherence to predetermined protocols and making data freely available. We, like everyone, are subject to the unwitting influence of our bias. The question is whether the Keller et al. publication of 2001 manifests unconscious bias or deliberate misrepresentation.

The original and restored studies, the study data, reviews and

> *responses are all available at* study329.org, *offering a broad range of options when it comes to consideration of authorship, research misconduct and the newly described species, "research parasite."*[152]

In her conflict of interest declaration linked to the Keller response, Gabrielle Carlson, a well-regarded researcher at Stony Brook University, declared research support from Pfizer and GlaxoSmithKline. In response to a question about the company's role and whether it had any role in study design, data collection, access, analysis, interpretation, writing of the report or the decision to publish, she wrote, "Stony Brook was a site in the two projects. The studies were industry-sponsored FDA-requested trials over which the company had complete control. We merely supplied patients." This drew the following tweet from Carl Elliott featuring a photo of a dump truck:

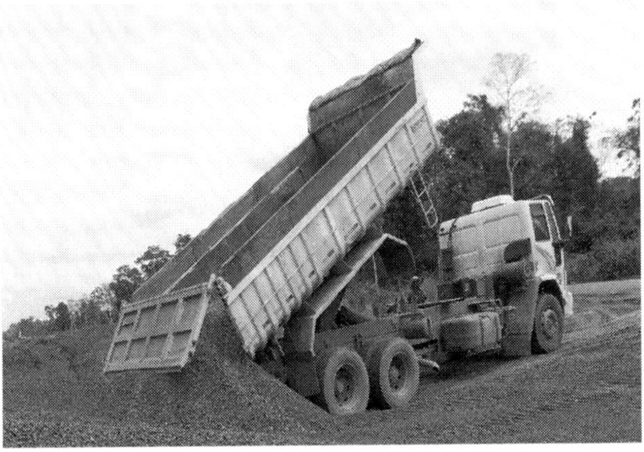

"We merely supplied the patients". *The statement on this disclosure form, by one of the authors of the notorious Study 329, pretty much sums up what's wrong with today's industry-sponsored, multi-site clinical trials. HT @RxISK*

CHAPTER 14

Son of 329

At a meeting of the British Association for Psychopharmacology in London in 1997, which Healy chaired, Stan Kutcher and Rachel Klein indicated that Study 329 would be the first to look at the longer-term outcome of treatment. However, when the Keller paper appeared, there was only an acute eight-week phase.

When GSK put the Clinical Study Reports up on its website in 2004, it became clear there was a CSR for the acute phase of the study and another for the continuation phase. The protocol described the objectives for the continuation phase as follows:

- To provide information on the safety profile of paroxetine and imipramine when these agents are given to adolescents for an extended period of time;
- To estimate the rate of relapse among paroxetine, imipramine, and placebo responders who were maintained on treatment.

The continuation phase "was not designed to determine whether paroxetine or imipramine are superior to placebo in preventing relapse," but instead "to provide information on the relapse rates of responders over an extended period."

After writing up the acute phase of Study 329, before GSK withdrew access to the periscope, RIAT set to work on the continuation phase data. Their work has resulted in a published paper[153], the full text of which is available on *study329.org* along with all reviews.

A key element was knowing what to do about the taper phase. Those who dropped out at the end of the acute phase went through taper, as did those who dropped out in the continuation phase and those who made it to the end of the continuation phase. Working out what do in each case involved scrutiny of the case files. This was not something that could be done from the CSR combined with Appendices A–G. The team presented the data in several ways in the paper, one of which is by duration of exposure. Some reviewers objected to this—but this was how Lilly, GSK and Pfizer had presented the suicide data in 1990 and 1991 when attempting to hide the problems of suicide.

Another problem was that many patients who were doing very well dropped out at the end of the acute phase—mostly among those taking placebo. Two thirds of the placebo dropouts were doing well when they dropped out, and two thirds of those who dropped out while doing well were on placebo. This raises doubts about the blind, which in some cases was clearly broken. One option is to regard these as potential completers. The Table below reflects this.

Another key factor was working out whether to designate as a relapse a patient who had a severe adverse event and for instance attempted suicide. The RIAT team opted to do so.

These are the headline findings from the continuation phase paper:

- relapses were higher on paroxetine than on placebo—Table 1
- efficacy is indistinguishable between treatments—Figure 1
- the taper phase of the study is the riskiest—Figure 2

Table 1: Rates of Response, Relapse, and Non-Response

	Paroxetine (n = 93)	Imipramine (n = 95)	Placebo (n = 87)
Response at some point	61	57	47
Completed responders (+ potential responders)	15 (+3)	12 (+1)	12 (+9)
Lack of efficacy: acute phase	29	36	38
Lack of efficacy: continuation phase	3	2	2
Acute phase dropouts	9	16	14
Continuation dropouts	12	14	11
Acute phase relapse	6	5	3
Continuation phase relapse	19	10	7
Total relapses	25 (41%)	15 (26%)	10 (21%)

Figure 1: Treatment Effectiveness

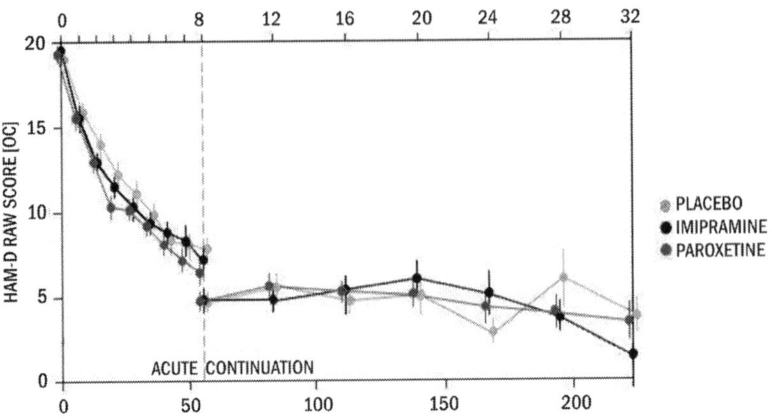

Figure 2: Behavioural events per 100 weeks exposure for acute, continuation and taper phases

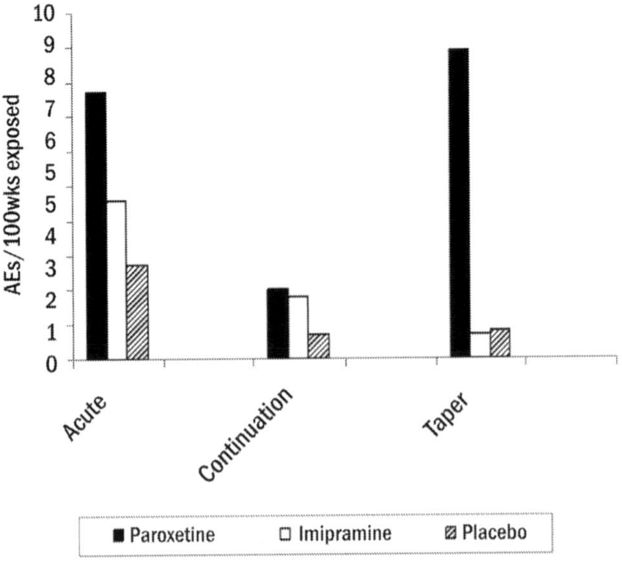

From the paper

The original Study 329 investigators are to be commended for undertaking a study that included a continuation phase for the purposes of providing longitudinal data on the treatment of adolescents with major depression. As one of the few bodies of data offering information on longer term treatment of adolescents with mood disorders, the study data are of value.

We analysed and reported the continuation phase according to the original Study 329 protocol. We draw minimal conclusions regarding efficacy and harms, inviting others to offer their own analysis.

The number of patients relapsing was designated a secondary outcome in Study 329. The results, however, remain unpublished. In our analysis, although we used more stringent criteria (i.e. remission) for response, we found higher rates of response in all three treatment groups than were reported in Keller et al. or in the text of the CSRs prepared by SKB, because we followed the classification in the CSR Appendix D, where response is based on HAM-D scores only, regardless of whether the patient or doctor violated the protocol.

Our analysis revealed more relapses in the active treatment groups than on placebo. This is in part determined by our decision to include in the relapse category patients who had a significant adverse event in the behavioral domain, but the higher numbers hold whether or not these patients are included.

Relapse was not a primary endpoint of the trial, and cannot be analysed in a way that would allow a definitive statement about rates of relapse compared to placebo. It can also be difficult to distinguish between apparent relapse and an adverse drug reaction, requiring caution in the case of patients who fail to respond to active treatment. Some of the patients in this study appear to have become paranoid or manic, or to have had a depressive relapse, all of which might lead to further diagnoses and/or prescriptions (a prescribing cascade) when in fact the wisest course of action might be to withdraw treatment.

The data on adverse events controlled for duration of exposure points to the taper phase as the riskiest period of treatment. It was difficult to be confident of the exact duration of exposure in the taper phase in some patients, but our estimates of duration are not likely to have inflated adverse event figures.

The CSR argued that simply looking at relapses is not a good way to establish long-term comparative efficacy. It proposed a randomized discontinuation design as the best way forward. However, the data from this study point to a discontinuation syndrome associated with paroxetine use. If this is the case, a randomized discontinuation design would not work, and we would be left with a more naturalistic option like the present study.

With regard to adverse events, the continuation phase of the study stands out as a phase where fewer adverse events either happened or were recorded. This is not surprising. It might be expected that the acute phase would weed out those patients not suited to the treatment they were on. But simple explanations like this may not fully account for the data, in that the patients entering the continuation phase appeared to have as many adverse events during the acute phase as those patients who did not opt to continue with treatment.

There are no other studies in this age group that we are aware of with which this study can be compared.

In our reporting of the acute phase of Study 329, we suggested that researchers and clinicians should recognise the potential biases in published research, including the potential barriers to accurate reporting of harms to which this study pointed. We also urged regulatory authorities to mandate access to trial data. This analysis of the continuation phase of Study 329 adds further weight to this recommendation.

It also adds weight to our invitation to others to access the data we have used. We are very clear that the analyses offered here are not the only ones possible. Our understanding of this dataset can only be enhanced by input from others who may make differing calls regarding coding and/or apply different analytic tools to the data.

Testing *JAACAP*

When the acute phase was written up, *BMJ* expressed interest in have it. Another option had been to test *JAACAP*. The continuation phase gave the team a chance to exercise this option.

The submission went to *JAACAP* on March 16, and the authors had a response from Andrés Martin by April 27, with five anonymous reviews and a note: "Thank you for the opportunity to consider your manuscript. I append below the comments from five peer reviewers. I regret that based on these critiques, and on my own careful consideration of your paper, I cannot accept it for publication."[154]

Two of the reviewers were favourable: "I do think that this paper is well written, and I also think that it provides meaningful additions to the literature. The data are clearly novel." "My general impression is that many passages could be edited to more concise form… In general, the tables seem to be a tedious listing of data. I offer no alternative; perhaps this is the best that can be done.

The team had made it clear that there were many more tables than was needed but that we were offering the reviewers as much data as possible. If accepted the number of tables could be trimmed.

One review was mixed and two were less favourable. A theme among these reviewers was that they wanted to be told what the data meant. Rather than be given tables of side effects data, they wanted the data to be handled statistically so that they would only have to consider any data that were statistically significant. It is inappropriate, however, to use statistics for harms when the data were not collected systematically.

Reviewer 3 was most exercised, but seemed to be reviewing the acute phase paper rather than the continuation phase:

> *You published a previous article in which you purportedly debunked the acute trial, drawing exactly the opposite conclusions from the original authors: not efficacious, with an increase in harms rather than well-tolerated and effective. This amazing feat set me to reading the original article and your re-analysis of the acute trial as well as the exchange of letters, besides the current manuscript. That homework brought the following realizations:*
>
> - *The conclusions hinge on what aspect of the data one attends to. E.g., The original authors chose to disregard their originally chosen 2 primary outcomes and instead attend to 4 secondary outcomes that most clinicians would agree validly reflect depression outcome, concluding effectiveness (poor science but clinical common sense). You chose to disregard those secondary outcomes that showed benefit even though one of them (Ham-D <8) was closely related to one of the original primary outcomes and another (CGI-I) was one of the pre-specified secondary outcomes, and instead rigorously followed the primary outcomes specified in the protocol (accurate science, but clinically obtuse).*
> - *You were critical of the original report well before you saw the data and you set out to analyze it as a misreported trial; in other words, you were on a mission. This is OK in itself; clinical science advances by having open debates about alternative interpretations, which can generate testable hypotheses, but:*
> - *Both you and the original authors appear to have conflicts of interest that may have colored your choice of which data to attend to. They may have wanted to report a positive trial and appear to have had some research funding from the manufacturer of one of the drugs. You, on the other hand, profited (and continue to profit) from forensic consulting fees. It should be noted that any financial benefit*

the original authors had is long gone and was probably gone by the time of their publication (although professional pride may still be an incentive to defend the original conclusions), while you stand to profit in the future from more forensic work.

- *Your interpretation of the safety data benefits from hindsight but risks the hazards of second-guessing the judgment of clinicians who were on the scene. Since the trial was carried out, we now have a better appreciation of suicide risk than was extant then, and you were able to apply that updated knowledge. On the other hand, it is risky (and not necessarily the best science) to reject what the original clinicians decided about attribution based solely on paper records without seeing the patient.*

But then, after more in this vein, this reviewer concluded: "This could be an interesting and provocative article, and you have clearly put a lot of work into mining the details, but you need to provide its context more clearly for readers."

However, Andrés Martin wasn't interested in giving the RIAT team a chance to provide more context. The team already knew that the likely home of the article was in the International Journal of Risk and Safety in Medicine whose editor, Chris van Boxtel, had been briefed about the detour through *JAACAP* with its aim of seeing how *JAACAP* responded.

The continuation phase of Study 329 saw the light of day in December 2016—19 years after the data collection had stopped.

CHAPTER 15

The Bitter End

On October 10, 2002, the FDA sent GSK an approvable letter, the first step in allowing the company to market Paxil to children and adolescents. The head of FDA's psychiatric drugs division at the time was Thomas Laughren.

Laughren worked at FDA from the mid-1980s to 2012. From the Prozac suicide hearings in 1991 to when he intervened to dismiss the apparent risk of suicidality on Zoloft in paediatric OCD trials, his role seems to have been to bat away concerns,

At the September 2004 Black Box Hearings, the public was allocated three-minute slots to make a pitch. People walked to a central well facing Laughren, Temple and Katz of FDA and the experts on the panel, including Robert Gibbons to speak. Mary Ellen Winter told the assembled room about her 23-year-old daughter Beth:

> *Beth was looking forward to a career in communication and was experiencing some anxiety and having trouble sleeping when she consulted our family physician. He prescribed Paxil and said she would start feeling better in two weeks. Seven days later Beth took her own life.*
>
> *We, like most of you in this room, grew up with confidence in the strides made in medicine and accepted with faith antibiotics and vaccinations prescribed. We believed the FDA would always act to protect our family's well-being. When my daughter went to our family GP last year, we trusted that our doctor was well educated and informed. We were wrong. We now know that pharmaceutical sales are a high-stake business, driven to increase shareholder wealth. The consolidation of pharmaceutical companies like GlaxoSmithKline has resulted in increased sophistication in the quest to market and distribute pharmaceutical products.*

> *Priority has moved from health to profit. Not all doctors are equipped to understand the marketing targets they have become. The FDA has allowed our daughter to be the victim of a highly commercial enterprise that selectively releases clinical data to maximize sales efforts and seeks only to gain corporate profits…*
>
> *As residents of the State of New York, we thank our Attorney General, Eliot Spitzer, for addressing issues that the FDA has been unwilling to address.*[155]

In the 72nd and second last slot Mathy Downing confronted Laughren:

> *On January 10, 2004, our beautiful little girl, Candace, died by hanging four days after ingesting 100 mg of Zoloft. She was 12 years old. The autopsy report indicated that Zoloft was present in her system. We had no warning that this would happen. This was not a child who had ever been depressed or had suicidal ideation. She was a happy little girl and a friend to everyone. She had been prescribed Zoloft for generalized anxiety disorder, by a qualified child psychiatrist, which manifested in school anxiety… She had the full support of a loving, caring, functional family and a nurturing school environment.*
>
> *Her death not only affected us but rocked our community… When Candace died, her school was closed for the day of her memorial service, a service that had to be held in the school gym in order to seat the thousand or so people who attended. How ironic, Dr. Laughren, that your family attended Candace's memorial service. Our daughters had been in class together since kindergarten. How devastating to us that your daughter will graduate from the school that they both attended for the past eight years and that Candace will never have the opportunity to do so.*
>
> *Candace's death was entirely avoidable, had we been given appropriate warnings and implications of the possible effects of Zoloft. It should have been our choice to make and not yours. We are not comforted by the insensitive comments of a corrupt and uncaring FDA or pharmaceutical benefactors such as Pfizer who sit in their ivory towers, passing*

> *judgments on the lives and deaths of so many innocent children. The blood of these children is on your hands. To continue to blame the victim rather than the drug is wrong. To make such blatant statements that depressed children run the risk of becoming suicidal does not fit the profile of our little girl.*[156]

Laughren vanished from FDA in December 2012.[157] To say he retired doesn't seem right. Many were left wondering at an abrupt exit, a few months after he had become acting head of central nervous system (CNS) drugs at FDA, replacing Russell Katz.

His departure triggered an outpouring of anger among patients, their families, and activists. Many of the references were in line with Hannah Arendt's evocation of the banality of evil. Almost immediately after Laughren vanished from the FDA, Pfizer wheeled him out as an expert witness defending it in a set of Zoloft birth defect cases.

Catch 62

On October 10, 1962, John F Kennedy signed a set of amendments to the U.S. Food and Drugs Act into law. Following the thalidomide catastrophe, these amendments put RCTs in place as the eye of a needle through which company drugs had to be threaded to get on the market. Drugs were risky. It was important they could be shown to work. A positive result in an RCT could stand as proof a drug worked.

This was a naïve move. The person responsible for writing RCTs into the regulations, Louis Lasagna, spent the rest of his career trying to undo the harm done. There is no better symbol of the Catch 62 he helped create than the fact that as of October 1962, only one drug had been shown to be effective and safe in a placebo controlled RCT before entry to the market—thalidomide. Lasagna was the person who ran the trial.

The new requirement for RCTs led to their industrial production. The mantra that RCTs offer gold standard evidence on drugs emerged quickly and has been used ever since to discredit the observations of clinicians and patients.

By the 1980s, there were enough RCTs in place for academics supported by Pharma to create evidence-based standards of care—guidelines. Up to the mid-1980s in both private and public health systems, costs had been contained by, and service development channelled through, medical discretion. Health-care administrators worked with medical and nursing staff who knew what the job involved. But guidelines transformed administrators into managers who no longer needed to rely on medical or nursing staff to tell them what was reasonable. The guidelines spelt out what worked

Better yet, managers and politicians had academics with a hand on the bible swear to them that even though the number one medication at the top of the latest standard of care might be the most expensive, health economics (invented by the pharmaceutical industry in the 1980s) had shown that its use would in fact save money in addition to delivering the best-quality health care. This was a managerial and political win-win.

Anyone who might protest would have to appeal against the standard of care. Where is the evidence base for doing what you think we should be doing doc? Claiming conflicts of interest on the part of those who drew up the standards is a weak card to play. Claiming the entire literature on which the standards were based was junk is a recipe for detention.

Study 329 is typical of all company trials done from the 1980s onward. It is trials like Study 329 that have been embodied in guidelines that dictate the medical treatments everyone now gets—whatever their age or condition.

In 2002, when *Panorama* began to investigate, there had been 70 Open Label studies, all claiming the newer antidepressants were wonderfully effective and safe in children and adolescents. RCTs are supposed to be a check on the clinical enthusiasm often found in Open Label studies. If the RCTs are negative, the scales are supposed to drop from clinical eyes and doctors are supposed to recoil from the latest snake oil.

In the wake of the 2004 Black Box hearings, it became clear there had been 20 RCTs involving close to 4,000 children—all negative, and all showing an excess of suicidality on treatment. All publications from these trials were ghost- or company-written. These RCTs didn't stop the drugs from being prescribed because all publications claimed the drugs worked well and were safe. This is the greatest known divide in medicine between what the data show and the academic literature claims.

Between 2006 and 2015, 15 more trials of antidepressants recruiting more than 6,000 children took place. All are negative and show an excess of suicidality on treatment. The trials continue because the six-month patent extension a trial gives is worth billions. Some recent trials with centres in the Russian Federation, Colombia and Mexico, along with foster homes and correctional facilities in the United States, make Study 329 look like a paragon of research propriety.

Against a background of over 30 negative RCTs, including 7 negative Prozac trials, prescribing antidepressants to distressed teenagers should have come to a full-stop but, while antidepressant use for teenagers briefly stalled in Britain, by 2018, aside from contraceptives, even in Britain antidepressants had become the most commonly prescribed drugs in adolescent girls generally.

Alongside this medication increase, there is a rising tide of admissions for self-harm, which is not what is supposed to happen when treatments work. It's not just antidepressant use that is rising in adolescents—it's all psychotropic drug use as antidepressant disinhibition or suicidality spun as bipolar disorder leads to treatment with anticonvulsants or antipsychotics.

As the prescription tide rose, the British Minister for Health in 2016 said children's mental health services were the greatest failing of National Health System. Services were failing despite more and more money being pumped in. The money is largely going into more screening, which picks up more children in distress with more ending up on treatment, and more auditors to ensure greater adherence to guidelines that still recommend SSRIs, in particular Prozac, and more managers to manage the deteriorating situation, none of whom are capable of recognizing, never mind tackling, the source of the problem. This is the best example there is of the vacuum at the heart of modern healthcare.

Aside from suicide, most psychotropic drugs affect the heart. Teenagers put on them, especially in combination treatments, drop dead.

Pretty well 100% of those who take an SSRI have an immediate genital numbing. For some this can persist for decades after treatment stops. Adolescents affected will be eunuchs.

Antidepressants cause dependence. Over 80% of antidepressant takers of all ages have been on them for more than a year, many for decades. For adolescents this is an extra problem as SSRIs inhibit growth, and cause weight gain, which affect self-image.

Women enter their childbearing years in adolescence. The evidence is compelling that SSRIs cause birth defects and autism spectrum disorders, and trigger miscarriages, which makes them a risk factor for future mental health problems. Women, dependent on their meds who know these drugs can harm their baby, face a difficult situation.

The problem for any prescriber faced with a distressed child is that the standard of care recommends using SSRI drugs. If on the basis of common sense or clinical experience, a nurse or doctor opts not to use these drugs and the family of the child are not happy or anything goes wrong, they will be questioned as to why they went against the standard of care and are increasingly likely to lose their job.

We get on the train

The difficulty for anyone inside or outside of medicine trying to get to grips with the problem now is that the playbook has changed. *Panorama* in 2004 could use the traditional media playbook—find an insider who reveals the scandal. This is a rotten apple in the barrel script, but we now face a rotten barrel. It focuses on one incident where a Jew or group of Jews gets beaten up on the streets of a German town, when the problem now is the evidence points to plans to remove the entire Jewish community from Greater Germany.

The default response from politicians faced with questions about things going wrong is to finger doctors prescribing off guidelines or off-label. The media help them do this by pitching the problems this way. This fiction works all too well because our natural inclination if things go wrong is to look for the person who is responsible. But we are now at greater risk from doctors who keep to guidelines than from doctors who don't, just as we once were from Germans who kept to the rules rather than from those who didn't.

A seemingly safe response for politicians or the media faced with evidence of a problem like antidepressant use in teenagers is to pitch for more money to be put into healthcare but into services other than drug services—in the case of distressed teenagers into counselling or therapy. This money will simply increase drug use.

The situation we now have turns many of the Good Guys like Medicins sans Frontieres (MSF), Doctors without Borders, the American Civil Liberties Union (ACLU) or even Churches into Bad Guys. By lobbying for access to medicines, claiming everyone has a right to drugs, including the latest drugs, they come close to being Pharma's best friends.

This lobbying was right in 2000, when it focused on access to Triple Therapy for AIDS in Third World settings. But there are almost no drugs developed since 1980 that save lives the way Triple Therapy for AIDS does. In pushing for access to antidepressants, statins, hypoglycemics and drugs for osteoporosis, and neglecting safety the Good Guys have become part of the problem.

As regards medical academics, there is some scope to view this story in Rip Van Winkle terms. Martin Keller and his colleagues were decent people. They certainly weren't out of the ordinary. When Study 329 began, they fell asleep in one kind of a world only to wake up in a different one, in which they were being deposed under oath. After their long sleep, despite other evidence of preserved cognitive faculties, Keller and Ryan had marked amnesia. The one person who seemed to have a good recall of what happened was Sally Laden.

But the way things have developed since make it's difficult to sustain the Rip van Winkle interpretation. Karen Wagner was the first author on Pfizer's studies of Zoloft in childhood depression and Forest's study of citalopram (study CIT-MD-18). Both were ghost-written. Forest were later fined by the Department of Justice, just as GSK were. While Study 329 was being published in the *BMJ*, with Wagner's role in focus for the American Association for Child and Adolescent Psychiatry (AACAP) members, including testimony that most articles her name was on were ghost-written, AACAP members voted her in as AACAP President. Given CIT-MD-18's serious flaws, Jon Jureidini, Jay Amsterdam and Leemon McHenry wrote to the editor of the *American Journal of Psychiatry* and Maria Oquendo, President of the American Psychiatric Association, suggesting it be retracted. There was no response.

Informed consent forms were introduced to drug trials in 1962. Their original purpose was to ensure everyone entering a trial of a new drug was informed that they were being asked to take an unapproved drug. Up till then doctors often tested out new drugs on people without letting them know. This development helped set up ethics committees and create the profession of bioethicists.

Skilfully over the next decades, drug companies changed the wording of these forms to include phrases to the effect that we will never reveal your data to anyone else. They now use the fact that participants have signed these forms to block access to the data from trials in which people have participated and in which they may have been injured. The consent form in Study 329 states,

> *I understand that I am not more likely to experience side effects as a result of my participation in this study than if I were being treated with paroxetine or imipramine in the usual manner*

The commonest adult dose of imipramine is 150 mg, and lower doses are often used. The children in 329 were treated with a minimum of 150 mg of imipramine and then titrated up to 300 mg if possible. This trial design looks like an effort to make imipramine look bad and paroxetine good by contrast.

The high drop-out rate on imipramine is consistent with this. Where were the ethicists while this was being put in place?

By 1997, GSK faced a statistically significant doubling of the rate of suicidality on paroxetine compared to the placebo in 329. Drug-induced suicidality will have put these children at increased risk of becoming suicidal from any cause in the future. Individuals reacting this way are far more likely than the average to have similar responses to other SSRIs and drugs like doxycycline and Accutane. Their relatives are probably at greater risk also. It is important for the self-image of their children and their future care they be made aware of the likely role of paroxetine in triggering these events. Even if the results of this trial were not conclusive in their own right, there was enough known at the time to debrief them properly.

To this day, GSK has made no overtures to any of those affected. They say it is not their place to intrude on the sanctity of the doctor-patient relationship, and they are leaving it to the doctors of those affected to decide what, if anything, these people should be told—when the doctors have painted themselves into a corner.

Unless there is outreach to patients injured in clinical trials, no-one should believe any company proposals about responsible access to clinical trial data. Claims about the need to protect patient confidentiality are based on concerns for the company's welfare rather than the welfare of anyone harmed.

Where are the ethicists or the lawyers in all this?

Those whom we expect to protect us all seem to have gone missing. The trains have arrived to take us East. Most of us get on the trains figuring that someone somewhere will recognize a mistake has been made and will sort things out before its too late. Leaving it to others to spot the mistake is no longer a sensible strategy.

Skin in the game

In 2016 and 2017, the FDA licensed a number of new skin drugs including Siliq, Otezla, Taltz, and others. These anti-inflammatory drugs are aimed at a psoriasis market. The trials had been done in clinical trial mills in Ontario and elsewhere with the data inaccessible and the study publications ghostwritten.

There was a high rate of suicidal acts in these studies. Company spokespeople, aka doctors, claimed that psoriasis causes depression and this causes suicidal thinking.

But in fact, the labelling on these drugs mentions suicide more clearly than the labels for antidepressants did, and in the case of Siliq doctors can't prescribe it unless they take a course which tells them it can cause suicide. Pharmacists can't dispense it without taking a similar course, and patients can't get the drug without signing a form to indicate that they have been warned about these risks. So, if you were still wondering if drugs can cause suicide—they can.

They can also cause homicide. As early as 1994, the label for Pfizer's Zoloft, the brand name for sertraline, mentions reports of psychosis and violence on sertraline. The few doctors who read the small print of the label and might have noticed this will have thought, "Oh what a wonderfully responsible and transparent company Pfizer is, putting every single report they have even from complete nutters and Scientologists on the label—of course I'm not going to pay any heed to this."

In fact, Pfizer and other companies only mention these cases reported in to them when they can find no other way, no matter how desperately they try, to explain violence other than to make a link to Zoloft. There are well over 100 drugs, from close to every class of drug there is on the market, that contain similar mentions on their labels, including asthma drugs, cardiac drugs, anti-hypertensive drugs and drugs for hair restoration.

Emotionally labile student

In March 2012, a 24-year-old studying neuroscience at the University of Colorado who was socially anxious and somewhat obsessive went to a campus doctor and was put on a benzodiazepine and sertraline. A week later, he complained of memory problems in class, and the benzodiazepine was swapped for a beta-blocker. His memory problems continued, and the beta-blocker dose was reduced. Beta-blockers and benzodiazepines can cause memory problems. Both can also act as antidotes to the anxiety and agitation sertraline can cause.

Meanwhile the sertraline was increased from 50 mg to 100 mg to 150 mg per day.

- He began flirting in a way that was out of character for him.
- He began spending wildly, where he had been frugal.
- He began visiting dating sites, which he had never done before.
- He signed up for motorcycle classes without a reason to do so.
- He terminated his only friendship with a girl in an abrupt way.
- He began talking for the first time of violence.

One friend said, "He began to "loosen up a bit" on medication and "became more talkative to random people." In a notebook, he made clear he had lost his sense of fear and developed a "dysphoric mania." This is a good description of the emotional instability that SSRIs can cause—a state in which anyone affected can rapidly swing from feeling energized and reckless, to depressed and suicidal.

SSRIs cause sexual dysfunction. He had it. The higher the dose, the worse it became. Sexual numbing goes hand in hand with emotional numbing and this too was present and became more marked as the sertraline increased. His feelings were blunted.

Prior to sertraline, he had thoughts that it might be no harm to "nuke" the human race. Such thoughts are not uncommon in introverts and the socially anxious. He told his doctors about them, and it is clear that they didn't regard this as mental illness. But on sertraline, he began to think about specific homicidal acts. These new thoughts were entirely different to his former vague hostility. They were focused, specific and "realistic."

SSRIs can do this to anyone—even normal volunteers. People who have been suicidal in the past and who become suicidal on SSRIs can distinguish the new ideas from their usual ideas. Some can hold both sets of thoughts in their mind at the same time. In this case, he did not just have thoughts that differed from those he had had before—he had a different motivational link to his thoughts. There was now a possibility that he might act on these thoughts in a way he would never have done before.

He tried to tell his doctors what was going on. Their response was that he was responsible for his own thoughts and actions. In the face of people threatening to kill themselves and others, nine times out of ten this used to be the correct reaction for someone working in mental health—it reduces the risk of violence to others. It is not the correct reaction when treatment with an SSRI goes wrong.

He attempted to communicate the changes he was experiencing in messages to classmates, but no one knew him well enough to pick up on it. There are difficulties in conveying alien thoughts of the kind that can be triggered by an SSRI:

- Few of us think a drug could do something like this, making it difficult to make a link.
- At first when thoughts like these happen, no one knows how to manage them.
- With problems like this, we often communicate obliquely. We think we have hinted enough for others to understand what is going on, only to find they don't.

There are recognized difficulties in communicating the adverse effects of a drug to the doctor who has put you on the drug hoping to help you. When things go wrong, the doctor can seem like the only way out of the problem and no one wants to antagonize their doctor for this reason. Push too hard, and the doctor gets nasty.

He dropped out of college at the end of June 2012. After three months on sertraline, he stopped abruptly from a dose of 150 mg, unaware of the risks of dependence and withdrawal. Over the next three weeks, he became confused and even more emotionally labile. The emotional blunting and depersonalization that started on sertraline continued, as it can for months after treatment is stopped.

On July 20, 2012, James Holmes entered a movie theatre in Aurora, Colorado, showing a premiere of *The Dark Knight Rises* and, opening fire, killed 12 people and left 70 injured.

He was arrested and hospitalized. Four months later, he became disturbed in hospital and was prescribed a variety of tranquilizers. He was also put on another SSRI for the first time since the end of June, and five days later attempted to kill himself. Buried in his history was evidence that he had reacted to a serotonin reuptake inhibiting antihistamine in the past with agitation. After the killings, both his parents were put on SSRIs and reacted poorly with horrific dreams in one case and emotional blunting in the other.

From May to July 2015, Holmes stood trial. It was certain from the start he would be found guilty. The prosecutor was asking for the death penalty. His legal team wanted to save his life. They opted to play a mental illness card. But for the last-minute qualms of one juror, Holmes would have been executed. His defense was weak—he did not have a serious mental illness. Despite defence experts torturing every little personality quirk back to his preteen years, nothing could change the fact that before walking into a university clinic in March 2012 with social anxiety problems, Holmes was very average with no mental health problems. He ended up with 12 life sentences and 3,300 years in prison.

Simply from the basic narrative of his case, there was a drug defence. There were also compelling data from the trials in adolescents that Zoloft could cause violence. The trial data shows that while these drugs trigger suicidality in some, they increase the risk of violence in others who, like Holmes, are more anxious and introverted than depressed. In 2006, the Black Box Warning was extended to those up to the age of 25—Holmes was 24. But Holmes's lawyers found it impossible to grasp the treatment nettle.

Every treatment with a drug or combination of drugs risks producing a frenzy. When the confusion is gross, medical and legal systems feel able to blame the drug, such as when a person goes berserk within 48 hours of having the drug. Don Schell offers an example of this: after starting Paxil in Wyoming in 1998, he killed his wife, daughter, granddaughter and then himself. The Wyoming jury blamed the drug, not Schell. This is easier to do when the perpetrator is dead.

But with a person sitting calmly in court, a lawyer faces a formidable task. First, they must find a doctor able to make a case when almost no doctors have any expertise in establishing whether a drug has caused any adverse event. Few know how to marshal a drug-related argument, especially a behavioural event.

If she finds an expert, the lawyer then needs to shepherd a jury along a narrow ledge. Questioning a prescription drug is to question the entire system on which most of us believe our safety depends. To acquit Holmes, we have to find the entire system—academic journals that accept ghostwritten articles, experts who don't have the guts to ask for the raw data, regulators who are pressured by government to partner industry—guilty.

At the height of the IRA bombing campaign in Britain in the 1980s, four innocent Irish people were jailed after a pub bombing in Guildford. Several English people took up their case. The most senior judge in England responded, "If their story is right, it is such an appalling vista it cannot be. Wrongfully convicted prisoners should stay in jail rather than be freed and risk a loss of public confidence in the law."

Substitute "his" for "their" and you have the position James Holmes was in. For many, it is better for a Holmes to get executed than for us to lose confidence in those responsible for looking after us.

Most readers likely will figure they are a long way from Holmes's position or that of Irish people locked up in English jails. But if a treatment injures you or a member of your family, you will end up in the same position. If you attempt to find out what went wrong, you will find yourself up against a system that will almost certainly end up not just acquitting itself but perhaps even congratulate itself on having kept to procedures every step of which conformed to standards of care.

You may be offered condolences for a dead husband, parent or child but in the absence of procedures that include boxes for death by antidepressant, statin or antibiotic, the services you make enquiries of will not be able to account for the injuries or death. At best you will be offered some weaselly words about there being controversy about a possible link between antidepressants and suicide—or something comparable for other drugs and deaths. No-one in the hospital or service you or your family were treated in is going to make a call that yes in this case the antidepressant we put you on caused this death—because to do so would require service processes to contain boxes for these possibilities and how to manage them.

Today's doctors are better trained to break bad news, but not to hear bad news. Underneath the surface of many otherwise decent people in healthcare lies someone who thinks they are an expert and who, convinced of their own good intentions, figures the primary duty of the person who comes to them is to do as they are told. But how can anyone be an expert given the kind of knowledge that tumbles out of studies like Study 329?

Power and democracy.

Study 329 is a story of the greatest failure in medicine. But the same story can be old about almost all drugs and for people of all ages.

Pharmaceutical companies make chemicals. We are the laboratories in which medicines are made. Medicines are chemicals used for a social purpose—to treat conditions that we define as diseases. Drugs cannot come into being unless we as healthy volunteers and later as patients in clinical trials agree to take them to see what happens. Without our participation, there is no drug.

Our willingness to participate in these studies was born out of a sense of civic duty. We participated on the understanding that taking risks might injure us but would benefit a community that included our friends, relatives, and children. We did so for free—in perhaps the greatest-ever example of how a system geared to people rather than products can make economic sense. The system worked in the 1960s and extended the compass of human freedom from many epidemics and other scourges to which our ancestors had been subject for millennia, and which took a horrific toll of children's lives.

But the research in which we once participated has morphed from scientific studies whose data were in the public domain into company trials where the data have been sequestered. We are never informed about this sequestration of our data. We assume that we are participating in science, and that the data arising from the risks we take are broadly available to scientists, as they once were.

It would be an easy matter to remedy this—by ensuring that the consent forms for a trial tell us whether the company will sequester our data. The only trials that are not going to jeopardize the health and well-being of our friends, children and communities are ones where the data are fully available. Otherwise companies will parade "their" trials in which injurious side effects are hidden, artfully coded or simply eliminated. If doctors or the courts believe them, any effort on our part to seek redress will fail at the first hurdle.

Evidence-based medicine as first conceived was a highly moral enterprise. It takes courage to subject all our preconceptions to testing, and to then treat the people who come to us for care on the basis of the data. But what passes for evidence-based medicine now is a sham. We need to recover the perspective that science, far from being value-free, values data and does so with a passion. "Controlled trials" that involve restricted access to data are not science and following selected "data" can only diminish both caregivers and patients.

If all the data on the benefits and hazards of treatment were available, the exuberance that companies can engender by marketing agents of supposedly extraordinary efficacy and almost no risks would be curbed. And if it were curbed, the vast profits that support the most sophisticated marketing on the planet, conjures diseases out of vicissitudes and can reconfigure our very selves to suit its purposes would in some measure be tempered. If this happened, clinical practice would have a better chance of being something closer to what it should be—one person consulting another.

This is not just about the legal consequences of hiding data. Faced with a choice between believing you when something goes wrong on treatment or believing the scientific evidence, nine out of ten doctors will believe the "science." And possibly because they know there is something wrong somewhere, they will get nasty with you—sometimes extremely nasty. Many of us sense this and don't dare to raise the fact that the treatment is not suiting us. When you come up against it, it's like the Great White shark in Jaws appearing right beside your boat—a real shock.

At present, things are getting worse, not better. It's something doctors need to realize because if drugs work marvellously well and have no side effects, there are cheaper prescribers even more likely to keep to the guidelines. Unless doctors can make a case that their job is to bring good out of the use of a poison and that this requires a good and honest relationship between us and them, they will soon be out of business in all but name.

Postscript

On February 19, 2017, Mickey Nardo died. The first hint most people had that he was 1boringoldman was when his name appeared on the authorship line of "Restoring Study 329". After the paper came out, Emory University made him an Emeritus Professor of Psychiatry.

About the Authors

David Healy

David Healy is a psychiatrist, psychopharmacologist, scientist and author. He is now based at the Department of Family Medicine, in Canada's McMaster University. He is a co-founder of RxISK.org, an adverse event reporting website, and the co-founder of Samizdat Health Writer's Co-operative Inc. Healy's research covers treatment-induced problems, and the history of physical treatments in medicine. He has written more than 200 peer-reviewed articles, 200 other articles, and 24 books, including *The Antidepressant Era, Let Them Eat Prozac,* and *Pharmageddon.*

Joanna Le Noury

Le Noury is a psychologist, a physicians associate and Senior Research Fellow in Wales, who is the first author on the Restored Study 329, which became a citation classic almost immediately after its publication in 2014.

Julie Wood

With her husband Peter, Wood is the driving force behind RxISK.org, SSRI Stories and Study 329.org—a website that hosts all of the documents behind the Study 329 story. Like a growing number of others she lost a talented and beloved child to antidepressants

Acknowledgments

Peter and Julie Wood created the Study329.org website and in Julie's case put in a vast amount of time creating timelines for the website—material which shaped this book. The website hosts the Panorama programs as well as all interviews listed in the text and its timelines contain many of the key documents.

Our other authors on Study 329—Mickey Nardo, Melissa Raven, Catalin Tufanaru, and Jon Jureidini—with whom we spent two years under the thundercloud of a common experience will hopefully read this account of what happened with some interest. They will no doubt be acutely aware it is not authoritative and may well feel there is room for more than one account of what was an extraordinary two years.

Peter Doshi, Andy Vickery, Skip Murgatroyd, Cindy Hall, Leemon McHenry, Andy Bell, Shelley Jofre, Dee Mangin, Charles Medawar and Andrew Herxheimer were also central to moving the story forward. Without them the *BMJ* article and this book would not have happened. Others who contributed hugely include Sarah Boseley, Barney Carroll, and Johanna Ryan.

Where other journals like *BMJ* were scared of being sued, Chris Van Boxtel, the former editor of the *International Journal of Risk and Safety in Medicine,* Chris held his nerve and took more articles in this area than anyone else.

Many people within the pharmaceutical industry helped. There is probably more courage and integrity within Pharma than in healthcare.

Endnotes

1 For references supporting the portrait painted here see Healy, D. The Antidepressant Era, (Harvard University Press, Cambridge Ma 1997); and Healy, D. The Creation of Psychopharmacology, (Harvard University Press, Cambridge Ma 2002).

2 Smith MC, *A Social History of the Minor Tranquilizers* (New York: Haworth Press, 1991)

3 Medawar C. Interview on *study329.org*

4 Lader M, Interview on *study329.org*

5 Ayd F. Interview on *study329.org*

6 Delini-Stula A, Interview on *study329.org*; Waldmeir P, Interview on *study329.org*

7 Shepherd M. Interview on *study329.org*

8 Sandler M. Interview on *study329.org*

9 Ashcroft G. Interview on *study329.org*

10 Axelrod J. Interview on *study329.org*

11 Schildkraut JJ, Interview on *study329.org*

12 For more detail on this story see Healy D, *Let Them Eat Prozac* (Toronto: Lorimer / New York: New York University Press 2003).

13 Carlsson A, Interview on *study329.org*

14 Lambert P & CLRTP, Interview on *study329.org*

15 Pinder R, Interview on *study329.org*

16 Rapoport J, Interview on *study329.org*

17 Pedersen V & Bogeso K, Interview on *study329.org*

18 Coppen A, Interview on *study329.org*

19 Communication to Lilly U.S. from Lilly Bad Homburg by B v. Keitz, May 25, 1984, containing a translation of an unofficially received medical comment on the fluoxetine application to the German regulators.

20 Healy D, *Let Them Eat Prozac*, (New York University Press, New York 2004) p 36.

21 Bech P, Interview on *study329.org*

22 Medawar C, Interview on *study329.org*; Medawar C, "The antidepressant web", *International Journal of Risk & Safety in Medicine* (1997) 10:75–125.

23 Rosenbaum JF, Fava M, Hoog SL, Ashcroft RC, Krebs W, "Selective serotonin reuptake inhibitor discontinuation syndrome: a randomised clinical study," *Biological Psychiatry* (1998), 44:77–87. See also socialaudit.org.uk

24 Shepherd M, Interview on *study329.org*

25 Carlsson A, Interview on *study329.org*

26 Healy D, Savage M, "Reserpine exhumed", *British Journal of Psychiatry* (1998), 172(5):376–378

27 Healy D, Mangin D, Does my Bias look Big in This? In Baylis F, Ballantyne, A. eds., Clinical Research involving Pregnant Women (Basal, Switzerland: Springer 2016), 197-208.

28 Healy D, Le Noury J, Harris M, Butt M, Linden S, Whitaker C, Zou L, Roberts AP, Mortality for schizophrenia and related psychoses: data from two cohorts, 1875–1924 and 1994–2010, BMJ Open (2012), 2:e001810, doi:10.1136/bmjopen-2012-001810

29 Cole J, Interview on *study329.org*

30 King A, Riddle MA, Chappell PB, Hardin MT, Anderson GM, Lombroso P, Scahill L, "Emergence of self-destructive phenomena in children and adolescents during fluoxetine treatment", Journal of American Academy of Child & Adolescent Psychiatry (1991), 30:171-176

31 References to all these documents are available on *study329.org* in the SSRI Timeline as well as on healyprozac.com and in Healy, *Let them Eat Prozac.*

32 Beasley CM, Dornseif BE, Bosomworth JC, Sayler ME, Rampey AH, Heiligenstein JH, Thomson VL, Murphy DJ, Masica DN, "Fluoxetine and suicide: a meta-analysis of controlled trials of treatment for depression", *British Medical Journal* (1991), 303:685–692.

33 Deposition of Wilma Harrison in *Miller Vs Pfizer,* March 14, 2000.

34 Fergusson D, Doucette S, Cranley-Glass K, Shapiro S, Healy D, Hebert P, Hutton B, "The association between suicide attempts and selective serotonin reuptake inhibitors: systematic review of randomised controlled trials", British Medical Journal (2005), 330(7488):396–399, doi:https://doi.org/10.1136/bmj.330.7488.396

35 Healy, *Let Them Eat Prozac.*

36 Trial testimony from Nancy Lord in *Fentress vs Eli Lilly* (October 24, 1994).

37 Ibid., p. 49.

38 Ibid., p. 54.

39 Ibid., p. 52.

40 Schulz-Solce N. Trial testimony in *Fentress vs Eli Lilly* by video from deposition, p. 185. See also chapter 11 for relevant figures on suicidal acts.

41 In Cornwell J, *The Power to Harm: Mind, Medicine, and Murder on Trial* (New York: Viking, 1996), p. 286.

42 Ibid., pp. 286–287.

43 For more detail see Healy D, Herxheimer A, Menkes D, "Antidepressants and violence: problems at the interface of medicine and law," *PLoS Medicine* (2006), 3, doi:10.1371/journal.pmed.0030372

44 Medicines and Healthcare Products Regulatory Agency. It is Britain's equivalent of the FDA.

45 For the following quotes see SSRI Timeline, *study329.org*

46 Kuhn R, Interview on *study329.org*

47 Klein R, Interview on *study329.org*

48 BAP Meeting Transcript on *study329.org*

49 Emslie GJ, Rush AJ, Weinberg WA, Kowatch RA, Hughes CW, Carmody T, Rintelmann J, "A double-blind, randomized, placebo-controlled trial of fluoxetine in children and adolescents with depression", *Archives of General Psychiatry* (1997), 54:1031–1037.

50 Healy, *Let Them Eat Prozac.*

51 This letter and follow up correspondence are available on *study329.org*

52 The video and transcript of this program are available on *study329.org*

53 The video and transcript for "Emails from the Edge" are available on *study329.org*

54 Available on *study329.org*

55 Available on *study329.org*

56 Lane C, *Shyness* (New Haven: Yale University Press, 2007).

57 ACNP paper available on Timeline on *study329.org*

58 The full document is on *study329.org*

59 A transcript of the hearings is available on *study329.org*

60 Kondro, W. and Sibbald, B. "Drug company experts advised staff to withhold data about SSRI use in children", *CMAJ.* Mar 2; 170 (5), (2004) 783. https://www.ncbi.nlm.nih.gov/pmc/articles/PMC343848/

61 Lancet Editorial, "Depressing Research", *Lancet* 363, (2004), 1335.

62 "GlaxoSmithKline Settles Lawsuit with Spitzer", eCommerce Times, By Richard Casey, Aug 26, 2004

63 A video and transcript of the program are available on *study329.org*

64 A video and transcript of the program are available on *study329.org*

65 Emslie GJ, Rush AJ, Weinberg WA, Kowatch RA, Hughes CW, Carmody T, Rintelmann J, "A Double-blind, Randomized, A placebo-Controlled Trial of Fluoxetine in Children and Adolescents With Depression", *Archives of General Psychiatry* (1997), 54:1031–37.

66 Emslie GJ, Heiligenstein JH, Wagner KD, Hoog S, Ernest DE, Brown E, Nilsson M, Jacobson JG, "Fluoxetine for acute treatment of depression in children and adolescents: a placebo-controlled, randomized clinical trial", *Journal of the American Academy of Child & Adolescent Psychiatry* (2002), 41:1205–1215.

67 See Mosholder, "Medical Review of Prozac", 2001, on *study329.org*

68 March SS, Petrycki S, Curry J, Wells K, Fairbank J, Burns B, Domino M, McNulty S, Vitiello B, Severe J, "Treatment for Adolescents With Depression Study (TADS) Team, Fluoxetine, cognitive-behavioral therapy, and their combination for adolescents with depression: Treatment for Adolescents With Depression Study (TADS) randomized controlled trial", *JAMA* (2004), 292(7):807–820.

69 Hogberg G, Antonnucio D, Healy D, "Suicidal risk from TADS study was higher than it first appeared", *International Journal of Risk & Safety in Medicine* (2015), 27:85–91, doi:10.3233/JRS-150645

70 Ibid.

71 To view letter go to Background, timeline, 2002, Oct 10, at *study329.org*

72 Transcript for this program is on *study329.org*

73 Weller IVD, Ashby D, Brook R, Chambers MGA, Chick JD, Drummond C, Ebmeier KP, Gunnell DJ, Hawking H, Mukaetova-Ladinska E, O'Tierney E, Taylor RJ, York A, Zwi M, *Report of the CSM Expert Working Group on the Safety of Selective Serotonin Reuptake Inhibitor Antidepressants* (June 2003).

74 To view Clinical Review document go to Background, timeline, February 1, 2004, at *study329.org*

75 Kirsch I, *The Emperor's New Drugs* (New York: Basic Books, 2010).

76 Lenzer J, "Drug Secrets: What the FDA isn't telling", *Slate Magazine* (September 27 2005).

77 A transcript of these two days hearings is on *Study329.org*

78 To view letter go to Background, timeline, September 23, 2004 "Statement of Robert Temple, M.D., Director, Office of Medical Policy, the FDA", at *study329.org*

79 Program and transcript available on *study329.org*

80 *Report of the CSM Expert Working Group on the safety of selective serotonin reuptake inhibitors 2004.* www.mhra.gov.uk/home/idcplg?IdcService= GET_FILE&dID=1391

81 Healy D, *Let Them Eat Prozac.*

82 Comment (October 1, 2008) by Lawrence Diller MD, Walnut Creek, CA, on Gibbons et al., "SSRIs, adolescent suicide, and the Black Box: lingering questions", *Psychiatric Times* (October 1, 2007).

83 American College of Neuropsychpharmacology, "ACNP issues final report on SSRIs and suicidal behavior in youth: task force finds urgent need for effective treatment for depression in children and adolescents " (November 23, 2005).

84 Verkes RJ, Van der Mast RC, Hengeveld MW, Tuyl JP, Zwindermann AH, Van Kempen GM, "Reduction by paroxetine of suicidal behavior in patients with repeated suicide attempts but not major depression", *American Journal of Psychiatry* (1998), 155:543–547.

85 Update April 5th 2006, Paroxetine Adult Suicidality Analysis. gsk.com/media/paroxetine/briefing_doc.pdf

86 GSK 2006 Press Release.

87 To view the GSK "Dear Health Care Professional" letter go to link at *study329.org*, Background, timeline, see link at May, 2006

88 U.S. Department of Health and Human Services, Food and Drug Administration (FDA) Centre for Drug Evaluation Research (CDER) Psychopharmacologic Drugs Advisory Committee (December 13, 2006). To view transcript go to link Background, Timeline, Dec 2006, at *study329.org*

89 U.S. Food and Drug Administration, "Antidepressant Use in Children, Adolescents, and Adultsæ (May 2, 2007), www.fda.gov/Drugs/DrugSafety/InformationbyDrugClass/UCM096273

90 Gibbons R, Brown CH, Hur K, Davis J, Mann JJ, "Suicidal thoughts and behavior with antidepressant treatment: reanalysis of the randomized placebo-controlled studies of fluoxetine and venlafaxine", *Archives of General Psychiatry* (2012), 69(6):580–587, doi:10.1001/archgenpsychiatry.2011.2048;

91 Gibbons RD, Hur K, Brown CH, Davis JM, Mann J, "Benefits from antidepressants: synthesis of 6-week patient-level outcomes from double-blind placebo-controlled randomized trials of fluoxetine and venlafaxine," *Archives of General Psychiatry* (2012), 69(6):572–579, doi:10.1001/archgenpsychiatry.2011.2044

92 1boringoldman blog, April 14 and 15, 2012, 1boringoldman.com

93 Lu CY, Zhang F, Lakoma MD, Madden JM, Rusinak D, Penfold RB, Simon G, Ahmedani BK, Clarke G, Hunkeler EM, Waitzfelder B, Owen-Smith A, Raebel MA, Rossom R, Coleman KJ, Copeland LA, Soumerai SB, "Changes in antidepressant use by young people and suicidal behavior after FDA warnings and media coverage: quasi-experimental study", *BMJ* 2014; 348: g3596 doi: 10.1136/bmj.g3596

94 For Rapid Responses to Lu et al – see Study 329.org

95 Fiddaman B, Kelly Posner Gerstenhaber — incredulous!, Fiddaman Blog (May 25, 2017), https://fiddaman.blogspot.co.uk/2017/05/kelly-posner-gerstenhaber-incredulous.html#.WYRiY4jyvIV

96 Note: references for most of the material and documents in this chapter are available at *study329.org* (see Background, Requests to retract original Study 329) and in Jureidini J, "Paxil study 329: paroxetine vs imipramine vs placebo in adolescents," *Healthy Skepticism* (January 2010), www.healthyskepticism.org/global/news/int/hsin2010-01

97 Weintrob A, "Paroxetine in adolescent major depression", *Journal of American Academy of Child and Adolescent Psychiatry* (2002) 41(4): 363.

98 Parsons M, "Paroxetine in adolescent major depression", *Journal of American Academy of Child and Adolescent Psychiatry* (2002), 41(4): 364.

99 Keller MB, Ryan ND, Wagner KD, "Paroxetine in adolescent major depression (reply)", *Journal of the American Academy of Child & Adolescent Psychiatry* (2002), 41(4):364.

100 Correll CU, Pleak RR, "Paroxetine in adolescent major depression (letter to editor)", *Journal of the American Academy of Child & Adolescent Psychiatry* (2002), 41(11):1269.

101 Keller MB, McCafferty JP, "Paroxetine in adolescent major depression (reply)', *Journal of the American Academy of Child & Adolescent Psychiatry* (2002), 41(11):1270.

102 Silveira R, Jainer AK, Singh R, "Paroxetine in adolescent major depression (letter to editor)", *Journal of the American Academy of Child & Adolescent Psychiatry* (2002), 41(11):1270.

103 Jureidini J, Tonkin A, "Paroxetine in adolescent major depression (letter to editor)", *Journal of the American Academy of Child & Adolescent Psychiatry* (2003), 42(5):514.

104 http://www.healthyskepticism.org/files/docs/gsk/paroxetine/study329/Dulcan.pdf

105 Jureidini J, Tonkin A, "Paroxetine in major depression (letter to editor)", *Journal of American Academy of Child and Adolescent Psychiatry,* (2003), 42(5):514

106 Keller MB, Ryan ND, Strober M, Weller EB, McCafferty JP, Hagino OR, Birmaher B, Wagner KD, "Paroxetine in major depression (reply)", *Journal of the American Academy of Child & Adolescent Psychiatry* (2003), 42(5):514-515.

107 Keller M, "Keller deposition", *Beverly Smith vs. SmithKline Beecham,* (September 6, 2006), redacted version on *study329.org*

108 Laden S, "Laden deposition", *Beverly Smith vs. SmithKline Beecham* (March 15, 2007), redacted version on *study329.org*

109 Scientific Therapeutics Information, Inc (STI) (2006) www.stimedinfo.com (see McHenry and Jureidini, 2008 below).

110 McHenry LB, Jureidini J, "Industry sponsored ghostwriting in clinical trial reporting: a case study", *Accountability in Research* (2008), 15:152–167.

111 Keller MB, Ryan ND, Strober M, Klein RG, Kutcher SP, Birmaher B, Hagino OR, Koplewicz H, Carlson GA, Clarke GN, Emslie GJ, Feinberg D, Geller B, Kusumakar V, Papatheodorou G, Sack WH, Sweeney M, Wagner KD, Weller EB, Winters NC, Oakes R, McCafferty JP, "Efficacy of paroxetine in the treatment of adolescent major depression: a randomized, controlled trial", *Journal of the American Academy of Child & Adolescent Psychiatry* (2001), 40(7):762–772.

112 British Broadcasting Corporation (BBC) "Secrets of the drug trials, Panorama" (January 29, 2007). Full transcript of the Jofre-Dulcan interview available on *study329.org*.

113 Jureidini J, McHenry LB, Mansfield PR, "Clinical trials and drug promotion: selective reporting of Study 329", *International Journal of Risk & Safety in Medicine* (2008), 20:73–81, doi: 10.3233/JRS-2008-0426

114 Pinder R, Interview on *study329.org*

115 Jureidini JN, Jureidini ES, "226 Papers/Letters that Cite Keller et al.'s Report of GlaxoSmithKline's Study 329 of Antidepressants for Adolescents" (February 2008), www.healthyskepticism.org/files/docs/gsk/paroxetine/study329/Keller01Citations_000.doc

116 Jureidini J, McHenry L, "Conflicted medical journals and the failure of trust", *Accountability in Research* (2011), 18(1):45-54. Doi:1080/08989621.2011.542683.

117 See Requests to retract on www.*study329.org*

118 Vickery A, Interview on *study329.org*

119 Murgatroyd S, Interview on *study329.org*

120 Menzies KB, Interview on *study329.org*

121 For depositions see *study329.org*

122 Nemeroff C, Interview on *study329.org*

123 Keller M, deposition and personal accounts on *study329.org*

124 Schatzberg A, Interview on *study329.org*

125 Healy D, *Let Them Eat Prozac*

126 Nemeroff CB, Owens MJ, "Treatment of Mood Disorders", *Nature Neuroscience* (2002), 5:1068-1070, doi: 10.1038/nn943.

127 Peterson M, "Undisclosed financial ties prompt reproval of doctor", *New York Times* (August 3, 2003), www.nytimes.com/2003/08/03/us/undisclosed-financial-ties-prompt-reproval-of-doctor.html

128 Carroll B, Rubin R, "Editorial policies on financial disclosure". *Nature Neuroscience* (2003) 6:999-1001, with response by Nemeroff C, Schatzberg A.

129 Nemeroff CB, Mayberg HS, Krahl SE, McNamara J, Frazer A, Henry TR, George MS, Charney DS, Brannan SK, "VNS therapy in treatment-resistant depression: clinical evidence and putative neurobiological mechanisms", *Neuropsychopharmacology* (2006), 31:1345–1355.

130 Armstrong D, "Medical reviews face criticism over lapses," *Pittsburgh Post-Gazette* (from Wall Street Journal) (July 19, 2006), www.postgazette.com/pg/06200/706933-114.stm

131 Carey B, "Correcting the errors of disclosure", *New York Times* (July 25, 2006), www.nytimes.com/2006/07/25/health/25news.html

132 Nemeroff CB, Mayberg HS, Krahl SE, McNamara J, Frazer A, Henry TR, George MS, Charney DS, Brannan SK, "Corrigendum: VNS therapy in treatment-resistant depression: clinical evidence and putative neurobiological mechanisms", *Neuropsychopharmacology* (2006) 31:2329, doi:10.1038/sj.npp.1301190

133 Belanoff JK, Rothschild AJ, Cassidy F, DeBattista C, Baulieu EE, Schold C, Schatzberg AF, "An open label trial of C-1073 (mifepristone) for psychotic major depression", *Biological Psychiatry* (2002), 52:386–392

134 Stotts B, "Gadfly or watchdog? Accuracy in Academia" (July 15, 2008), http://www.academia.org/gadfly-or-watchdog/

135 Barney Carroll catalogued the evolution of this in a series of "Health Care Renewal" Blog posts that can be accessed on *study329.org*

136 "Preemption's requiem in the wake of WYETH V. LEVINE" (November 2016), www.baumhedlundlaw.com/pharmaceutical-articles/preemptions-requiem-wake-wyeth-v-levine/

137 http://articles.latimes.com/2008/oct/04/science/sci-doctors4#

138 Gøtzsche P, Interview on *study329.org*

139 *BMJ* (June 22, 2013), 346:23–26.

140 "Experts propose restoring invisible and abandoned trials 'to correct the scientific record'", *Science Daily* (June 14, 2013).

141 For the full correspondence between the RIAT team and *BMJ* during this submission process, along with the responses from the *BMJ* reviewers in their entirety, see *study329.org*

142 Winter C, "MedDRA in clinical trials—industry perspective", *SFDA-ICH MedDRA workshop*, Beijing (May 13-14, 2011), anyflip.com/hxlp/pijg/basic www.meddra.org/sites/default/files/page/documents_insert/christina_winter_2_meddra_in_clinical_trials_industry_perspective.pdf

143 http://www.legalweek.com/legal-week/news/2284819/ropes-gray-takes-lead-role-gsk-probe-into-china-bribery-claims

144 Le Noury J, Nardo J, Jureidini J, Healy D, Raven M, Aba-Jaoude E, Tufanaru C, "Restoring Study 329: efficacy and harms of paroxetine and imipramine in treatment of major depression in adolescence", *BMJ* (2015), 351:h4320, doi:10 .113 6/bmj. h4320

145 See United States Ex Rel. Greg Thorpe, Et Al. Plaintiffs, v. Glaxosmithkline Plc, and Glaxosmithkline Llc, Defendants, www.justice.gov/sites/default/files/opa/legacy/2012/07/02/us-complaint.pdf

146 Basken P, "Landmark analysis of an infamous medical study points out the challenges of research oversight", *Chronicle of Higher Education* (September 17, 2015), www.chronicle.com/article/Landmark-Analysis-of-an/233179/

147 Linden, D, "Re: Restoring Study 329: efficacy and harms of paroxetine and imipramine in treatment of major depression in adolescence (rapid response)", *BMJ* (September 22, 2015), www.bmj.com/content/351/bmj.h4320/rr-9.

148 For all the rapid responses post publication of "Restoring Study 329" see *study329.org* or http://www.bmj.com/content/351/bmj.h4320/rapid-responses

149 Longo DL, Drazen JM, "Data sharing", *New England Journal of Medicine* (2016), 374:276–277, doi:10.1056/NEJMe1516564

150 Keller MB, Birmaher B, Carlson GA, Clarke GN, Emslie GJ, Koplewicz H, Kutcher S, Ryan N, Sack WH, Strober M, "Re: Restoring Study 329: efficacy and harms of paroxetine and imipramine in treatment of major depression in adolescence: Response from the authors of the original Study 329 (rapid response)", *BMJ* (January 18, 2016), www.bmj.com/content/351/bmj.h4320/rr-27

151 Doshi P, Jefferson T, "Response to Keller et al. re: RIAT", *BMJ* (January 20, 2016), www.bmj.com/content/351/bmj.h4320/rr-28

152 Jureidini JN, Healy D, Nardo M, Raven M, Abi-Jaoude E, Tufanaru C, Le Noury J, "Re: Restoring Study 329: Response to Keller and selected colleagues", *BMJ* (February 3, 2016), www.bmj.com/content/351/bmj.h4320/rr-29

153 Le Noury J, Nardo J, Healy D, Jureidini J, Raven M, Tufanuru C, Abi-Jaoude E, "Study 329: continuation phase", *International Journal of Risk & Safety in Medicine* (2016), 28:143–161.

154 For full copies of the *JAACAP* reviewers responses see study329

155 "Joint meeting of the CDER Psychopharmacologic Drugs Advisory Committee and the FDA Pediatric Advisory Committee", Bethesda, MD (September 13, 2004), p. 332.

156 Ibid., p. 435

157 "Controversial FDA official Tom Laughren retires", *BioSpace* (December 7, 2012), www.biospace.com/News/controversial-fda-official-tom-laughren-retires/281586

Index

Printed in Great Britain
by Amazon

41704481R00158